WHAT ARE YOU LOOKING AT?

I0118141

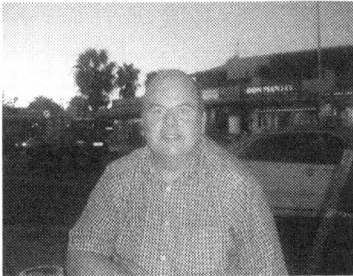

By Wayne Hadfield

"One million people commit suicide every year"
World Health Organisation

Published by:
Chipmunkapublishing
PO Box 6872
Brentwood
Essex
CM13 1ZT
United Kingdom

http://www.chipmunkapublishing.com

THINGS NOT TO DO

There are certain things I know not to do,
Make a list to remind myself to give a clue,
No more bottling things up inside,
No more putting things away a place to hide,

Not to get in touch with family that won't help me,
I have to keep contact going, so I'll be free,
From guilt that I've carried around for so long,
Why should I feel guilt, I've done nothing wrong,

This illness I have, is no fault of mine,
Think yourself lucky that you feel fine,
Do I regret having this condition, some days yes,
But it's who I am; I always try my best,

Four years ago things seemed great, no worries at all,
But were they that good, perhaps I needed to fall,
To realise what I'm really like, to find the real me,
Well four years is a long learning curve, to find my destiny,

Sometimes I'm hard on myself; I feel I've let you all down,
But you say I'm better than I used to be, good to be around,
So I'll tell you how I am each and every day,
I'll get over any obstacles that get in my way.

ONE YEAR FROM NOW

If I had a crystal ball to see myself a year from now,
What could my best be, could I look and say wow,
Just to feel proud of myself that would be great,
No more negative thoughts, move forward it's not to late,

Plenty of smiles, tears of laughter and of joy,
Back to living life in the fast lane a grown up boy,
Lots of music being played out loud and long,
Singing my heart out to whatever is my favourite song,

To feel happy in every single thing I do,
Keeping myself busy no time to feel blue,
Being free to say or do whatever I please,
Having no tension, feeling relaxed and at ease,

To be in touch with friends that I've let slip,
Being in control, coping with any small blip,
Giving help to people is something I'd like to do,
I've learnt so much, I could pass on to a few,

Going to bed each night knowing I've done my best,
Feeling proud that I've passed life's hardest test,
Having a feeling of contentment, happy to be me,
I would have the greatest feeling of being free.

ROLLERCOASTER

My head seems to be spinning around and
around,
So hard to keep my feet on the ground,
When things start to go well, how long will it last?
Forever haunted by a ghost from the past,

To be free from my ghost is that too much to ask,
Things seem so hard even a simple task,
Takes its toll on me, I tire so quick,
I have a bad taste in my mouth I feel sick,

Sick and tired no end to this fight,
Why do some people say you look alright?
I don't look any different I've not gained a second
head,
Would you prefer it if I stay in bed,

I can draw from strength something inside,
I'm not going away I'm not about to hide,
Why should I this can happen to anyone,
But I'm determined to have some fun,

So as the rollercoaster goes up and down,
That's how my life is don't frown,
I'm always going to try my best,
And pass this long life time test.

<u>COULD THIS BE THE LAST TIME</u>

Could this be the last time I'm ever here,
A place where I've had to deal with my real fears,
Somewhere that's become like a second home,
Hours, days and weeks spent wondering as I
roam,

Thinking how things could and would be only if,
I've become a stronger person finally I've learnt
my gift,
Times when I've thought I'll never make it through,
But you've always stood by me, that's what makes
you, you,

Let's try to move forward a small step each day,
Getting over any obstacles that might get in our
way,
Were able to hold our heads high because were
so strong,
Together now forever it's taken us so long,

I believe everything happens for a particular
reason,
Let's hope we've now moved into our get well
season,
We've always had faith that things would turn out
right,
Whatever happens from now on everything's in
our sights,
So let all our prayers be answered from the man
above,

Together now and forever with our everlasting love.

MR RELAXED

I don't think I've ever known someone so calm and
at ease,
Nothing's ever too much trouble you always aim to
please,
The pleasure and hope you give comes straight
from the heart,
You inspire me not to finish but to make a new
start,

You make me feel safe, at peace with myself,
Helping everyone leaving no one on the shelf,
Remembering everyone's name giving it that
personal touch,
Going that extra mile nothing ever seems too
much,

Having a heart of gold not one made of glass,
Sharing all your wisdom, well your different class,
You've helped so many people in your unique
way,
Helping us to move forward each and everyday,

So please be proud of everything you do,
Because you've helped me so much, God bless
and thank you.

DRUG CULTURE

Your drug culture has caught up with you,
Not knowing fact from fiction, what's a lie what's
true?
Thinking you're in a different world you know that
can't be,
Walking around blindly not seeing what others can
see,

Life's one long party but you know it has to end,
No one really cares about you a pills your only
friend,
What do you gain from losing yourself if you don't
know who you are?
Not knowing what your boundaries you've pushed
your limits too far,

Stop for a minute and take a reality check,
Get off that slippery slope, you'll fall and break
your neck,
I suppose it's your choice, and you're free to
choose,
But have you anything to win, you've so much to
lose,

Quit while you can take your lifeline,
Live in reality with what you've got tell them this is
mine,
Then your fantasy can become your reality,
Moments that you've lost will regain there
normality,
No one laughs with you but at you don't you know,

Paper over what you want but the cracks still show.

I THOUGHT

I thought you were a friend, how wrong was I,
Our paths crossed, horns locked tell me why,
You called me something I can't forgive,
Don't tell me how I should live,

I know you are ill but so am I,
You pushed the wrong button so don't lie,
Do what you must that's up to you,
But my knowledge is better; you don't have a clue,

I've stood up for you, told people you were nice,
Where did that get me I'm paying the price?
You've given me hassle, hassle I don't need,
I've never questioned your colour or creed,

If you'd had the trouble I'd had would you know,
Just to leave me alone, let me go,
I kept out of your way, so let me be,
Don't try and talk or get friendly with me,

I'm usually tolerant but I'm not going to be with
you,
Don't look at me, or you'll get what's due,
Not violence but a piece of my mind,
Then you'll have no one to hide behind.

FAITH

My faith is something that's personal to me,
It's what I have inside not for others to see,
I can't tell you about it, you wouldn't understand,
I suppose it just came to me nothing I had
planned,

When times have been bad my faith sees me
through,
It stays with me when I'm at my lowest, down and
blue,
I don't preach to people on how they should be,
I wouldn't dare do that so don't tell thee,

With this illness I have I've gained some insight,
Some power from above has given me guidance
and light,
Unless you've been there it's so hard to explain,
I suppose it's one of the perks for all the pain,

I hope I can stay focused and remain strong,
Any bad times I have won't be there for too long,
With faith on my side and your love too,
Good times are around the corner there long
overdue.

WHO AM I

Going back to somewhere I've spent so much time at,
Seems so strange quite surreal, fictional not fact,
It felt odd and I felt outcast and strange,
I was feeling jumbled up needed to be rearranged,

Faces were familiar, but had I moved on?
It was kind of weird a false situation,
I guess I'm hoping, that I can put things in the past,
Then any bad memories can fade and won't last,

You could say that it's become a bizarre second home,
Having spent so much time there, time spent alone,
So much time to have things spinning around in my head,
Lying there crying and shaking alone in my bed,

So lets hope that this is all left behind me,
To move on and make sure I'm the best I can be,
But I must remember to be careful and take my time,
Not feeling guilty because mental illness is my only crime,

In the future there's so much for me to do,
I should make a list, of not too many, maybe just a few,

Then I would feel a sense of pride of what I've achieved,
Make the most of my talents that I've received,

So I'll raise a glass celebrate what I am,
Have my life in order, my own mapped out plan,
To go on a journey that's full of fun,
Being born again a time to move on.

COULD THIS BE IT

I can see the light flickering for me,
My future seems a bit clearer a new destiny,
They say all things happen for a reason,
Perhaps I'm going into my get well season,

It seems that the change I want is on its way,
I must take my time; listen to what you say,
I know what I want but can I get it?
Re arrange my life, step by step, bit by bit,

For more than three and a half years now one
long learning curve,
Can I keep it together do what I must keep my
nerve?
To be the person I know that I can,
A better human being a born again man,

You see I have my faith one that's my own,
I won't preach to you I'll reap the seeds I've sown,
I know that I've got my god on my side,
I'll show you what I can achieve, show my pride,
So don't let me look back no more regrets,
I know deep inside of me that this is it.

SON OF MINE

Oh son of mine don't feel any shame,
What's happened to me, well you're not to blame,
I'm so proud of you how you handle things,
I hope I've had all the bad luck my condition
brings,

In you I would love to forfil my dreams,
Dreams that I've had taken from me hear my
screams,
Will you promise me you'll remember good times
we've had,
Don't think of me of always being depressed and
sad,

Years have come and gone oh so fast,
Fears you have won't always last,
You're growing up to be a fine young man,
The sky's the limit do all you can,

If you never try you'll never know,
Just how far you can go in life give it a go,
Don't be frightened, be strong you won't fail,
Your going to be king of the jungle alpha one
male.

TURNING THE CORNER

I think I've taken a turn in the right direction,
I can see light at the end of the tunnel my
homeward bound station,
I hope I'm not counting chickens before they've
hatched,
But I'm hoping that my doors been left off the
latch,

I've got a sort of tingling feeling inside,
One that's kind of feels good, one I mustn't hide,
It's overdue because I've been here for so long,
I'm desperate to get home, because that's where I
belong,

Things here are starting to get to me,
But I must stay strong try to keep my sanity,
I know that people are really ill and don't
understand,
Their own illness seems to be beating them
getting the upper hand,

But some seem to like being trapped in here,
They say they don't but what I've seen is so clear,
It's the way they act when staff are around,
But when on their own their true selves are found,

Surely things on the outside have to be better than
here,
Perhaps I'm missing something not seeing what's
clear,
I just wish I can stay out here forever,

But that's maybe a bit naive never say never,

So if the corner has been turned that's great,
Times a great healer, the waits worth the wait,
Just to be honest with myself that's all I can do,
Maybe I am to be one of the chosen few.

LOVE ME FOR WHO I AM

Love me for who I am,
Don't remember me as a broken man,
I wish there was something I could do,
To give you what's long overdue,

I know that you've all been in a position,
That's uncomfortable because of my condition,
I'm sorry for the way I've been,
And the ugly side of me that you've seen,

I know that I should've looked after you,
You showed me love kindness in pure form and
true,
I'm proud of you all in so many ways,
Let's live for today leave all our yesterdays,

If there's some thing I can pass on,
Is that you can handle any situation?
Your so courageous genuine and brave,
I can't thank you enough for the love you gave.

GOD LET THIS BE IT

Please god let this be it
A turning point bit by bit
I'll try to be good make it right
Something more than hope this special night,

Let me move on leave the past behind
Let me do my bit for all mankind
I'm going to be a better man
I've got my own special plan,

I must make up for time that's gone
A fresh start a new me has begun
Have I passed this mental test?
Please let me be my all time best,

I want to start to live life
To the full with no more strife

Be glad that I'm alive
No more falls or dives
Get myself well and ultra fit
So please god let this be it.

THE REAL ME

This is a story I hope comes true,
Like being re born a new me for you,
I feel like a monster is on the outside,
Your first impression of me, oh I wish I could, hide,

I'm sad to say that I'm ashamed of what I've
become, but with hard work and dedication could
it be undone?
I feel as a person that I've become so weak,
No confidence, no self esteem, maybe mild and
meek,

If I'm honest I know I'll never be how I was,
In some ways that's good, but things have been
lost,
If I could turn back time what would I change?
Maybe it's just impossible for me to try and
rearrange,

Just to feel happy is not too much to ask for,
Maybe in time there may be some miracle cure,
To put the last four years behind me and to move
on,
Reshuffle the cards I've been dealt and reposition,
Surely I'm not asking to much am I?
Please god help me, please hear my cry.

YOUR DAY OF REST

So the day you wanted has finally come,
There's a chill in the air, and a low sun,
You made an impact on me, one I won't forget,
That I couldn't help you is something I regret,

We lived so close from the same neighbourhood,
Now you've moved to a different level I'm sure it
will be good,
I've cried for you because I guess I know how you
feel,
But the events of two weeks ago seem so surreal,

It's the system that let you down; I guess you
slipped through,
Maybe with some proper help and care you'd find
the real you,
Please be at peace now, because it's what you
need,
Rest be safe and sound, rest with lessons you
heed,

Be free from all the crap that you carried around,
Make as much noise as you want without making
a sound,
Feel pride because you did what you thought was
right, I'll see your personality in the stars at night.

MY ILLNESS

If I could explain my situation would you understand?
You see my illness is in my head I fall into a band
People try to ignore us because they are so naive
If I let you in my head you might not believe

My illness is bipolar (also known as manic depression)
Please let me explain my situation
You see I get mood swings both high and low
How much can you understand?
I will explain and let you know

When I am high I feel like some kind of super human being
No worries in the world confidence brimming
Feeling careless and carefree nothing can bother me
Knowing what to do and see comes oh so easily

When feeling high I get the feeling of immortality
I may cause a scene but I don't care if people stare at me
I am convinced that nothing is wrong and I am just great
This won't last long so I have to get help before it's too late

It seems so cruel when you feel so good it has to end

So this condition is a life long demon and a good friend
Then following on as sure as night follows day
My mood drops really quick and I go the other way

Without too much of a warning sign
My mind switches and my mood declines
Just a feeling of utter desperation
I plunge into the depths of severe depression

People say what have you got to be depressed about
This gets me so annoyed makes me want to shout
There is no particular reason for how I am
I just wish I had a get well plan

WAITING GAME

How much longer do I have to wait?
Things need to get better it's not to late,
To get my life back on track,
No more trying to paper over the cracks,

A time to show courage, a time to show strength,
To take a few risks, but not at any length,
If I knew what to do I'd do it now,
I've got to make it through somehow,

The weeks go by with no change at all,
Feels like I'm banging my head against a brick
wall,
I sit and watch others come and go,
But I have to learn to let my true feelings show,

People say how can you be low when you have so
much,
But what I have doesn't change how I am such is
such,
Sometimes it's hard to put up a front,
I have to soldier on survive this mental hunt.

MISSING YOU

Why did you do it had you finally reached the end
We knew each other fairly well I would call you a
friend
I have cried a lot of tears I have felt so low and
blue
I will fight on for the cause but I am missing you

Unless you have been through a similar thing no
one can know
What thoughts we hide inside and what we can
show
I hope things can change for the better for the few
But you will always have a place in my head and I
am missing you

Why do the good ones have to go God seems so
unkind
There never seems much justice with those left
behind
I hope that you are at peace now, show me a sign
give me a clue
Because no matter what you did I am going to
miss you

I wish that I could turn back time make things
alright
But that's not going to be possible it's a wonderful
thing insight
So for now you are in my thoughts your peace
was long overdue

God bless you and goodbye I am really missing you

WHY AM I WRONG?

I know this illness affects us all,
Why is it me banging my head against the wall?
You say that I'm nasty well it's not what I think,
Leave me alone let my own ship sink,

It's like my freedoms been taken away from me,
My life's laid out naked for the entire world to see,
How can I look to the future with hope in my soul?
When each and every minute this illness has got a
hold,

I'd write a goodbye note but I don't want to go,
It's hard to shake the feeling when I'm so low,
Think of tomorrow, but that never comes,
I'm ashamed of this worthless person I've
become,

I feel so restricted nothing to live for,
I know it's a dead-end street my face on the floor,
I feel dirty ashamed no longer a man,
If I can't be who I want to be, then what point any
future plan?

I have so many emotions going on inside,
I need more help, but can't swallow my pride,
Forever feeling guilty, what have I done wrong?
Start the final record for one last song.

FEAR

Why do I have this fear when I am not scared?
Do I know secrets should they be shared?
Am I unique or do others feel the same?
Is my life one long reality game?

When will I know when the time is right?
To reveal all my strengths and all my might
Can I unlock the labyrinth in my mind?
Should I shut it away be cruel to be kind

Why does my mind need mending if it's not broke
Is God getting me to feel like some kind of joke?
Why do I feel guilty when I have tried my best?
Is this my life examination some kind of test?

No real answers for me just the same old question
I will lay myself bare I am open to your
suggestions
Are my happiest thoughts just blanked out?
Is the time right for me to scream and shout?

So who knows what my future holds
Will I die with stories untold?
Can I be remembered long after I have gone?
To look after everyone start what I have begun

REMEMBER

What do I remember from my childhood days
Let me try to reflect, I'll try to amaze
How would it be if I could change things
I live my life like songs that everyone sings,

I can recall my early years like a record collection
Have a brief look through and make your selection
You see music has always been a part of me
It's helped me keep some kind of sanity

Songs always mean different things to me
Places I've been, what I'd wished I could be
I remember lots of songs that make me laugh and
cry
Or sometimes I do both, for what reason, why?

You can interpret lyrics to your own situation
Let them inspire you, take you to your destination
Let your mind escape and be free
Always try to maintain your dignity

I remember nights singing and dancing away
Sorting out what would be the next record to play
3 minute hero, or a message to you
Or something played by Deacon Blue

I would have a favourite to play over and over
again
Knowing each word and note to perfection
keeping me sane
I would buy several records each and every week

Spending all my money on records to keep
Over the years my music knowledge grows and grows
All kinds of emotions provoked and it shows

KNOWING YOU

You think you know someone, how they appear,
But opinions change all is not clear,
You're not the person I thought I knew,
Are you ill or is what I'm seeing the real you,
If you've a problem with me please let me know,
You've let down your guard, the cracks do show.

You walk round like you own the place,
But the way you talk to people is a disgrace,
You moan about people, but you're the biggest
moaner of all,
One day you'll get what you deserve, a great big
fall,
If you're as clever and as smart as you think,
Why when you try to walk on water, you always
sink?

The plans you have change each and everyday,
But I'm smarter than you I remember what you
say,
One day you slag someone off, the next day
they're great,
I'm always polite to you, but don't call me your
mate,
The illness you have is the same as mine,
But I can behave, I can tow the line.

In a week you state that you'll be free,
But don't build your hopes up there's no
guarantee,

What you want is not always what you get,
You've told me things, that ill never forget,
Everyone's glad when you've passed by,
Perhaps open your eyes ask yourself why.

I might be wrong in my opinion of you,
So if I am then an apology is due,
But I'm sure I've seen the real man,
If you can be called a man, then anyone can,
So know I've said my peace, I'll leave you in
peace,
My chastation of you will know cease.

ISOLATED

Why is this illness of mine so isolating,
Tired of it all, fed up with waiting,
For things to take a turn for the better,
No more waiting for a welfare letter,
To tell me that I'm going to be fine,
To somehow mend my broken mind.

If you say I'm strong, why doesn't it feel?
That I'm so weak, my scars won't heal,
If I start to get better how would I know?
What would the signs be, how would it show,
Would I have a natural smile on my face?
Instead of one that feels out of place.

Surely it can't go on year after year,
Not getting well is my greatest fear,
Not being able to do the things I want,
Not through the lack of trying, just that I can't,
Why was this illness given to me and not you?
No one has the answers, not even a clue.

So many questions, but scared to ask,
Just such a heavy burden, a hard task,
The pressure is so intense it's so difficult to cope,
I have to carry on there's got to be hope,
Twenty one years now and still it goes on,
Sick to death of a life on medication.

Is my destiny here in my own hands?
Or am I so dependent on others for my plans,

So frustrated, no longer do I have dreams,
No one sees my internal crying, shouting and screams,
Everyone tells me to be patient, it takes time,
Why do I feel a prisoner, when mental illness is my only crime?

NORMAL

What is normal could you please explain?
Is normal being free from this mental pain?
Can I survive in this state I'm in?
Or does everything have to change, where would
it begin.

It's to do with an imbalance in my brain
With chemical changes again and again
It can't be cured just the symptoms treated
My engines gone wrong it's over heated

Refer to the manual what does it say
A complete overhaul then sent on my way
To hopefully cope no matter what
If I had been a lame horse I would have been shot

Does the answer lie in a packet of pills?
Or left alone could I cure my ills?
I question your professional ways of doing things
But I trust you to make changes with me nagging

The trouble is not two of us are the same
Getting it right is part of the game
But when you are alone who can you turn to
No one knows what we are going through

So from the outside what do you see?
I hear you say he looks fine to me
But I will swap with you for just 1 day
Then you would know what it's like to feel this way

FRUSTRATED

If I don't kick up a fuss, where will it leave me
Tortured, frustrated and drowning in my
uncertainty
I think that sometimes you don't think I exist
But I'm not going away I promise you this

Your meant to look after me, so why?
No one's around to see me shaking, to see me cry
Try to be more positive that's the way
But please don't ignore me I'm not going away

Why don't you remind us that's what they say
But it's your job not mine, for once earn your pay
What is it to you if it takes an extra week
Don't verbally abuse me, I'm no mental freak

Don't look as if your afraid of me
I'll do things my way and keep my dignity
So if I tell you something I expect you to hear
The more I explain it will become more clear

This illness is with me every single day
But I'm running on empty some would say
When my backs up against the wall just watch out
I'll come out fighting, you'll hear me shout

Yesterdays history, what's gone has gone
Today lets make the most of it love everyone
Tomorrow never comes, that's saying is true
But if it does, will it be for the chosen few

WHO

Running around you don't know where to begin
From the outside you're like a headless chicken
You eventually will go on empty and run out of gas
Make the most of it now because it just won't last

You claim to have a heart of gold
But you just think of yourself you soon turn cold
Why do you think that the world revolves around you?
Change your ways be to yourself be true

When you're good you're a nice person to know
But when you kick off see how people turn and go
They are not scared of you but they keep out of your way
How can you not listen to what other people say?

Knowing what you have to do and doing them are different things
If you don't play by the rules you know what that brings
So surely the decisions you make need to change
Shake yourself up and try and rearrange
Deep down you are no different to me
It's just harder for some people to see

SCARED

You ask how I am, to tell you how I feel
I suppose I keep so much inside not wanting to
reveal
The pain I feel is so intense, hard to explain
I don't want to go through all of it again

The trouble is I don't know what to do for the best
I've tried my hardest I think I'll leave it to the rest
To make decisions to make sure that it's right
Being able to get my head rested every night

Uncertainty seems all I have in my life right now
I've got to pull through but I don't know how
How will I plan my future when I can't live for today
Can I turn things around and be positive in the
things I say

The frustration I feel gets worse every day
I could tear down walls if I could pave a way
To help me get well what do I have to do
I'm so dependent and rely so much on you

So my illness is hidden it's so hard to tell
I might look normal but boy am I unwell
It will take as long as it takes so I have to wait
Try to be patient and not to get irate

I'll try harder to communicate and tell you how I
am
Because you care so much more where other's
don't give a damn

I know you can't fully understand what I'm going through
But I know your trying because that's you

BORN AGAIN

If life begins does that mean I'm born again?
If I'm born again, am I free from mental pain,
To be able to leave so much in the past,
Leaving everything behind, moving on fast,

To find myself with a new personality,
Is that what I need, what will be, will be,
I suppose that's too much to ask for,
I'm just uncertain, frightened and insecure,

Do I have the will power for the fight ahead?
Or should I isolate myself and stay in bed,
Would I get better or get better from that,
What's best for me so I can stay intact?

I feel like I'm walking along life's high wire,
Trying to extinguish my self made fire,
So how do I stop this raging inferno?
Does anyone have the answer, because I don't
know

So can I stay positive to keep myself a float?
Can I not get shipwrecked stay on my lifeboat?
Not knowing whether to sink or swim,
But prepared to take a gamble, maybe I can win,

I suppose I've got nothing left to lose,
I'm sick and tired having the permanent blues,
This cycle can't always go on it has to end,
Then I will be nearly fixed well on the mend.

<u>SO SO</u>

You ask me how I am; I tell you I'm so so,
I try hard to explain but can you ever know,
Could I get worse I didn't think I could,
To be honest and do all I know I should,

Taking more tablets will this be the cure,
Will it make me better or worse than I was before?
I have to be patient it's just a question of time,
But time stops for nobody especially my mind,

So if there's a formula one to make me well,
I'd like to bottle it, make it available and sell,
To everyone who's in the same boat as me,
Then there'd be no one shipwrecked with their
mentality,

Like a never ending circle where did it all begin?
When did the cracks appear, was it born from
within?
Could I have done things better, so my illness
would be less?
I can't answer that, there's no point trying to
guess,

I know what's wrong with me, I just don't know
why,
Why did it happen to me, and just passed others
by,
I hear people say to me, well your looking well,
But my illness is inside my head, not so easy to
tell,

So the emptiness and void is so hard to explain,
Is the loss of confidence something I can regain?
Will I ever be the person I want to be?
So I'm happy and fulfilled with my identity.

LIFE AS A JOURNEY

My life seems to be like a fairground
I will open up and show you the sights and sounds
If you walk in then you will see
What it's like living and being plain simple me

First the rollercoaster one second high the next
low
But when, why and how long I just never know
Sometimes it's like I am never coming down
Then I feel like I have gone deep underground

Next the maze of mirrors what can I see
Lots of reflections but not knowing the real me
Not knowing where to go or which way to turn
No real sense of direction but I am willing to learn

Perhaps next on the coconut shy
Being hit on the head and wondering why
Not sure if I am ready to take the fall
To stay upright or fall flat on the floor

Straight onto the dodgems hit from side to side
Always trying to avoid but having nowhere to hide
Battered and bruised taking hit after hit
Finally slowing down and entering into the pit

Last but not least the merry go round
Gently going up and gently going down
Perhaps with insight then you will see
How my life's fairground is for me

PUBLIC AND PRIVATE MASKS

Looking from the outside well what do you see?
Can you see right through my defences and see
the real me?
Or do you look at me and say there is nothing
wrong
But if I start to tell you it would take so long

You see my illness eats away in my head
It's not caused by physical pain or something you
have said
I don't know how I will be day to day week to week
If only it was as simple as turning the other cheek

If you could look inside my mind then you would
understand
That sometimes are great and others I am a
broken man
An internal battering but no bruises to show
Keep taking the medicine but the pain won't go

Try hard not to look back and live in the past
But my history is who I am my mould has been
cast
When looking forward to the future what can I see
But no one knows what will happen tomorrow
what will be will be

It would be so nice to live each day to the full
Achieving small goals no more days that are dull
Just to be happy with a smile on my face
Not feeling some outcast from the human race

To have some confidence to come back bit by bit
Instead of avoiding everything a social misfit
To resist the temptation to throw it all in
Could this be the day my recovery will begin

HOW IT IS

So tired of this battle but I must win
Always fighting the demons from within
Having the desire to fight and soldier on
No battle can be lost the war must be won

Time allows the scars to heal
But the pains still there the blows are real
I have been knocked down many times before
I pick myself up and get up off the floor

I dust myself down start over and over again
Not to be beaten by anything fight the pain
No prizes to be won in the contest ahead
Finally time to put this illness to bed

Start living feel like I am born again
Get my head sorted out don't go insane
Try to say my luck will change
I just need shaking up to be rearranged

I know I am not the only one
Who's gone through this so I have begun
To try and get motivated and turn the page
No more living in anger no more life rage

So stop worrying when there is no need to be
scared
Start planning ahead try to be prepared
Have peace of mind if I can
Stay focus and live to my life plan

OUTSIDE LOOKING IN

If I was on the outside with you looking in,
What you would see might alarm you but let us
begin,
From the outside everything is normal nothing
looks wrong,
But something inside eats away like some
barbaric song.

Each of us is unique, no two of us the same,
They say its no ones fault; no one is to blame,
So why do people turn away, that wouldn't have
before,
Is it that I'm damaged goods, with one almighty
flaw?

To be treated as an equal, that would be a start,
To stand in life's identity parade, not able to be
picked apart,
No more to stay quiet, I'm not going to go away,
Trying to move forward each and everyday.

We are the silent illness, but that's society's
choice,
But if we come together what a determined voice,
No longer to be muted, no more shameful fear,
An uprising will be started, everyday and every
year.

So no more ignorance, you will be made aware,
It's up to you to change your ways to show us that
you care,

So whether I'm very high or very low and blue,
Just be oh so very weary, that this could happen
to you.

TRUTH & HONESTY

When darkest days are raining down on me,
Two things I must remember, be true with
honesty,
Even if the truth is hard, it's what I have to say,
By being like this I can make it through the day.

I can see that small ray of light, flickering for me,
Will I have in my own hands, my life's destiny?
To move on now, not being afraid to fall,
I must restart life's engine, if ever I should stall.

I believe what I've been through is one long, life
exam,
If I pass or fail, don't matter, what I am,
I hope to come through this much better than
before,
Be stronger, wiser, and more confident harder to
ignore.

This illness is never, ever going to go away,
But it will not beat me; I will win, day by day,
Even on a bad day, I'll tell myself this will pass,
The depressed and flat feeling, won't always last.

Hopefully the good days, will become more the
norm,
Lovely sunny days ahead, forgetting the bad
storm,
So if I have one quote, one that works for me,
Is to live my life with truth and honesty.

POSITIVE ASSETS

Try to think of things I have rather than I have not
To think of the things I have to give not things I
forgot
Try always to look forward only briefly glancing
back
To get my life together to get back on track

People say I'm strong I suppose it's vaguely true
I am good at putting up a front that no one can see
through
I'm scared to let down my guard afraid of what you
might see
To show it how it is then you will see the real me

To say how I want to be rather than I am
To be free from illness is my long term plan
But to be the best I can live from day to day
Working through life's obstacles that get in my
way

At the moment I feel trapped not knowing how I
will be
Sometimes I feel like escaping from this insanity
But this is real things are happening to me now
To get through the bad times to make it somehow

So if you ask me what assets see me through?
I don't think I have many just a vital few
So if I open up my life's briefcase this is what you
will see

Someone never going to give up someone open true with honesty

FIRST AID KIT

What do I need to keep me well?
Let me think about it then I will tell
First on my list would have to be hope
Without having this I simply wouldn't cope

Even when I am down and feeling blue
There are several things I need to do
I have to talk be honest and true
Hopefully then bad times will become fewer and
few

A spoonful of confidence is what I need
Not too much not overfeed
Just enough to get through each and every day
So I am not too high or get carried away

If I had a higher self esteem
I wouldn't be just a one man team
Everyone who helps me would be in my side
Then I would feel good no need to hide

I need to get fit be healthy and strong
Just to get well and nothing going wrong
To be free from worries that would be nice
That would be valued but not at any price

So all these things will help me stay well
The only way of knowing well time will tell
To help me stay well bit by bit
Then I have got life's survival kit

SPRING

Spring time a new me a new you
A time to move on and not to feel blue
A new beginning things start to grow
Flowers that were hidden begin to show

If my mind was like spring how would it be?
Could I start fresh and become a new me
Would I forget all my winter blues?
My mind would be free then I could chose

Start moving forward along life's highway
Straight through barriers that are in my way
Not looking back just forward that's me
Believe in my fate in life's destiny

Breathing in all things for the first time
Exhale bad memories and leave them behind
Move forward be strong and be true
Hope that bad days are fewer and few

Spring clean my mind that's what I will do
Remove all the clutter that's long overdue
Everything then is put in its right place
And bad memories can fade without a trace

LITTER

Life's like litter that's blown round and around
One moment flying up in the air then along the ground
To be picked up or left to rot
That was once useful is now easily forgot

I was once all new and was never used
But I got crumpled up my mind abused
My mind got scattered I lost the plot
I never asked for this illness I got

So will I get recycled and used again
To be well for years free from this pain
A new start a new me time to begin
Try to avoid being thrown in life's litter bin

So if I fall please help pick me up
If I am thirsty help me share your cup
If I am chucked away please help me be found
If I am muted could you be my sound

Help my mind be tidy let my life be litter free
Help get rid of my mind's rubbish that's hurting me
Let me be free to do all I have planned
Just simple things in life nothing to grand

FUTURE

What will the future hold what can I plan
Can my destiny be in my own two hands?
To start off take small steps day by day
Get over any hurdles that get in the way

Keep going forward never looking back
Try to keep going the right way around life's track
Don't be put off if I should fall
Brick by brick I can build that wall

You only live once or so they say
To be the best I can day by day
Live life to the full if I can
To be no more a broken man

Get fitter and stronger invent a new me
No need to drown in my own history
I will never forget who I am or where I am from
To be more humble share a love with everyone

In years to come I will look back at me
I am going to be so proud of what I see
Dreams fulfilled no stone unturned
To share with everyone life's lessons I have
learned

PERSONAL SHIELD

A shield of hope a shield to protect
A shield to welcome not to reject
Something to hide behind when things go wrong
Hopefully not to be used for too long

A family coat of arms to be worn by all
To be wrapped up in when we fall
Something to be shown off in all it's glory
A strong reminder of a never ending story

Think positive put bad memories away
Keep moving small steps forward each and every
day
The scars of battle are clear to see
A reminder to every one of what I claim to be

A flag of faith, colours true
Proud to be born under the red, white and blue
But all colours can fade into one
When a new age and era has begun

A motto simple to always stand by
A statement of fact, not a question why?
To pass down from father to son
Love, faith, hope and peace for everyone

My everlasting friend

My everlasting friend that's what you will be to me,
A special place in my heart for eternity,
The love you gave was unconditional and pure,
There's a big gap missing that's for sure,

Could I have done more to help you out?
You didn't cry in pain or give me a shout,
I tried so hard to take your pain,
But god called you; our loss is his gain,

I know that you're free now, to do as you please,
Running, jumping, playing, walking at ease,
I thank you for the great times we had,
Happy memories of you outweigh any hint of
being sad.

In memory of Maximus Hadfield (MAX)

2000-2005.

My valentine

I suppose it's a special time,
To you my love this valentine,
Without you oh where would I be?
Shipwrecked and deserted in the open sea,

Sometimes I don't express how grateful I am,
Having you as my wife, I'm a lucky man,
So my love for you gets stronger each day,
You help me over hurdles that are in my way,

Together, forever and never to part,
I love you so much with all of my heart,
You're my rock, my pillar, my statue of stone,
Your love's so strong I'll never be alone.

For Jane.

2005 THE YEAR AHEAD

2005 a New Year a new start
A time to move on but memories stay in the heart
Don't forget the past but try not to dwell
Start living in heaven and not a mental hell

2005 a year for dreams to come true
Throw out all of the old bring in all the new
A time to move forward in all walks of life
And not to fall back on a sharpened knife

Visions of laughter, fun and good times ahead
A time to start moving not stuck in bed
Try to stay focused be honest be true
So even the dark days are fewer and few

Hopes for the year are clear in my mind
Try to be more loving, understanding and kind
Be more positive even when feeling down
Straight from the heart and tears of a clown

There's light at the end of the tunnel
For each and everyone to see
But I have to be sure and certain
It's not an oncoming train aiming at me

Inch by inch and step by step
As time moves on the stronger I will get
One day at a time, week by week
Tell how it is no secrets to keep

Be the best I can each and every day
End each day by making myself say
Thank god I'm here and alive
And here's to a fantastic 2005

LIFE IS A JOURNEY

Life is a journey or so they say,
To drive straight ahead or to give way,
Round and around the roundabout leaving
different ways,
Living in the present not tomorrow or yesterday,

Take one step at a time arrive at the station,
Just buy a one way ticket, ride life's destination,
Head going fast winding down life's track,
Try always to look forward and never look back,

Fly away from it all leave the world again,
Let your head go on auto pilot relive the pain,
No more emergency landings be safe and sound,
Even at 30,000ft have both feet on the ground,

So tired of floating ship wrecked at sea,
Searching for that desert island in my own sanity,
Only games to win now, not to draw or lose,
Have a six month vacation on a fantasy cruise,

Forget my problems be an astronaut in space,
No one to answer to everything is in place,
Look down on the world with stars in my face,
Just one persons view on the entire human race,

Back down to earth with an almighty crash,
Lifeboats out stranded on my own survival raft,
Drifting alone just a blip in the sea,
Everyone is searching, reaching trying to rescue
me,

No one knows where life's journey will end,
But if I get lost an s.o.s. I'll send,
Whether found on land sky or sea,
What a one off journey my life will be.

WAITING

Am I waiting for something that might never arrive?
Things might not get better no matter what I try
You see I am good at putting on a brave face
But I can't help thinking I am a disgrace

This illness I have is so hard to explain
My own mental torture drives me insane
If you could see inside my head
You would be amazed that I got out of my bed

If it was as simple as pulling myself together
Then I would do it straight away that's not being clever
But I can't seem to pick myself up at all
I can live with the highs but I hate the falls

If there was a wonder drug then give me a shot
I assure you no one would want this illness I have got
I hear people say theirs some worse off
But that doesn't make me feel better I am paying the cost

So I guess I will have to dig deeper than I have done before
Hoping there is some kind of medical cure
A time when I can leave this in the past
Remaining well and happy is all I ask

Leave the past behind

The time is right to leave the past behind,
Wipe the slate clean; be cruel to be kind,
Move on to a newer and brighter dimension,
No more hanging in a mid air suspension,

What's gone has gone so why look back?
Keep looking forward on life's fast track,
Hold on to memories but try not letting them
dictate,
What my future holds for me well I'll have to wait,

Time stops for nobody, that's a simple fact,
So I must stay focused not let things distract
Me from being as good as I possibly can
Write things down so I can stick to a plan,

It's no good thinking of how things might have
been,
Or denying what's happened because it's to
obscene,
So from now on I must make a new start,
Go into things head on, just following my heart,
Try to put things to the back of my mind
Finally moving on leaving my past behind.

Sentimental

Certain songs always make me think,
Of how things could be, when I'm at the brink,
Not knowing what I'm fighting for,
Does anyone know a recipe for a miracle cure?

Is it possible to feel excited but also scared?
Things would be easier if no one cared,
People tell me I'm brave they tell me I'm strong,
But what if it's all a front could they be wrong,

Should I take my destiny take it with force?
Free myself from medication strangulation of
course,
If I fail there is no one else to blame,
Let me hold my head up high, without shame,

Others seem to be worse off than me,
But my pain is real; it's me with uncertainty,
It's me with all the answers, but has no questions,
Try what you will I'm open to your suggestion,
Be honest with me give me no bull,
Because I'm sick of feeling sentimental.

Tired

Not much sleep last night why,
Was my head racing if so why?
I thought I was relaxed and feeling good,
Have I crashed with an almighty thud?

Did I have too much on my mind?
Was something that was said cruel to be kind?
I know that I have to make a change,
Sort myself out try to rearrange,

Pains in my chest one thing after another,
Why can't I be well like any other?
I must get myself out of this trap,
To stop feeling altogether crap,

Surely I will get well this time,
I feel guilty when I've done no crime,
Honestly I don't bare anyone a grudge,
But don't disrespect me and try to judge,
Because if so I'll feel retired,
I'm so fed up of being low and tired.

DETOX MY MIND

Searching for clues don't know where to begin
To sort my life out throw rubbish in the bin
Detox my mind so the clutter has gone
A new age a new era a new time has begun

Leave all the crap that has been in my mind
Left in a place that I will never go and find
I suppose no one can tell me the future I will get
I might find out something I may well regret

I want to move on to give something back
Make a difference help people get on track
Pass on my experience tell people how it's been
Tell them what's worked for me I would be really
keen

My talking about mental illness barriers can come
down
It won't happen overnight but maybe given time
Mental illness will be treated just like any other
Out there in the open no longer under cover

2006 THE YEAR AHEAD

As a new year approaches it's a time for new hope
Pull on the resources I have to help me cope
Try to make a new beginning a new start
Not letting my head over rule my heart

A time to stay positive but realistic too
Hopefully bad times will become fewer and few
Looking forward to the future and whatever it
holds
Try not to be too cowardly be brave and bold

Sometimes a new year is a time to reflect
Thinking of things I should have done and not
neglect
But I suppose all I try is to make the most of any
situation
Then hopefully I can fulfil my dreams arrive at my
destination

What's gone has gone so try not to worry it can't
be changed
Start to put my house in order, tidy up and
rearrange
Then maybe 2006 will be the year for me
To find my true meaning and be the man I want to
be

HAPPY

Looking forward to a time when I can be happy
Surely it will happen soon I hope you will see
I know I can't go back to 4 years ago
Was I really happy then, well who knows?

To have laughter so much flying around
Feeling high but having both feet on the ground
Looking forward to be more socially free
To be good to be around, to be the real me

Having been depressed for nearly 4 years now
You can forget how to enjoy yourself feel guilt
somehow
You are scared if you see someone when you are
out
If you've a smile on your face they say what's that
all about

But I have done so much crying it's an emotional
outlet
I am not ashamed to admit with me what you see
is what you get
So if you see me looking happy it doesn't mean
everything is fine
It's my coping strategy one that's just mine

YOU LOOK FINE

You seem fine to me I hear you say
But looks are deceiving I'm masked every day
I hide behind it some say I do it too much
But that's how I feel such is such

Even when there are no tears I'm crying inside
I try to put on a brave face I've too much pride
But you know me and how I am
I don't like admitting that I'm a broken man

So if I'm broken so much how can I mend?
I've got my support network my survival friends
People who know me and who are always there
They tell me how it is show they care

To have a mental illness doesn't mean I'm mad
Think yourself lucky if it's something you have
never had
But you never know what's round the corner next
it could be you
Because it can come from nowhere out of the blue

LOOKING WELL

I hear you say hi you're looking well
But looks can be deceiving let me tell
How it is for me each and every day
Having this feeling that's not going away

Can you see the tears that I cry?
Do you wonder and ask yourself why
This is happening to me and not to you
What have I done wrong can you give me a clue

I can't move forward if I'm stuck in reverse
Why do I feel possessed feel like I've been cursed
It's hard to feel positive to see the way ahead
To feel the fright the fear and the dread

I am waiting for a sign of good days to come
Not always having the thoughts that I'm coming
undone
How long must I wait it seems so cruel
Am I the exception to the get well rule?

STOOD STILL

How can I move on when I'm always standing still?
Could I find a way to climb an endless hill?
What it takes is a small step at a time
But I cannot see those steps when the feet are mine

I'm told by everyone not to panic or to worry
But that's easier said than done I'm always saying sorry
I feel that I have let so many people down
My illness just seems to go around and around

I cannot change my past even if I tried
What has gone has gone and cannot be denied
So I will have to be the best I can each and every day
Try to get over any obstacles that get in my way

It's like climbing out of a very deep hole
You get so far out but can never reach your goal
So many small lifts but never quite enough
God no one tells you bipolar is so tough

The Four Seasons

Winter's here so cold and dark
Iced over puddles found in the park
Fill the air with frozen breath
Wrap up warm don't catch your death

Winter's here there's snow on the ground
Everyone's inside the house safe and sound
Winter nights seem oh so long
Everyday similar like a never ending song

But soon its spring so bright and clear
A new lease of life it's like a new year
Out in the countryside all green and blue
A lamb springs to life newer than new
Nights get brighter and longer too
A breath of fresh air for me and you

Then its summer the nights bright and long
People outdoors singing along to a song
The suns so warm and high in the sky
No time to worry or to ask why
People get into the holiday mood
Chatting and eating with their barbeque food

Then autumns comes leaves golden and brown
Strong winds blow them down and around
The nights get shorter dull and grey
Warning floods are on their way
Everyone starts to stay indoors
Another year over for seasons 1, 2, 3 and 4

Emotions

Lying in bed trying to sleep
Things spinning around secrets to keep
Could I tell could I explain?
Will my life ever be the same?

Some thoughts normal some are strange
Try to sort them out try to re-arrange
It's hard to explain the internal screaming
The pains still there even when I'm dreaming

So I will always be honest open and true
Try not to panic if one day I'm blue
Knowing the pain won't always last
No longer frightened by the ghost of my past

Take small steps day by day
Take the punches on the chin or dodge out the
way
I'm sure one day things will be fine
It's just that small question of time

So in the future how will it be?
When I look in the mirror whose reflection will I
see?
Will it be me slowly sinking and drowning?
Or standing proud confident not frowning

What will happen tomorrow well no one knows
But I want to stay focused and deal with the blows
And if I remain positive and strong
Then a wonderful journey comes join along

What's a New Year?

What's a New Year mean to me?
A time to put the previous year to history
A time to look forward not to look back
Think of the things I have rather than the things I
lack

To think of the things that is good to me
A kind loving and caring loyal family
Without them I would be nothing at all
I couldn't stand up on my own bound to fall

As a New Year starts can a New Year Begin?
Put out all of my old rubbish into the bin
To be positive but realistic too
Be honest to myself and to be true

Having my own faith one that's just for me
Can help me reach and fulfil my destiny
I must remember things I have learnt from my past
And the feeling of being the real me might last

Nobody knows how I will be in the year ahead
But if I can hold on to hope there will be less for
me to dread
Once again I will be able to hold my head up high
To enjoy a year every moment as it goes by

HAPPY DAYS

Happy Days so many when I was young
Not any warning signs of anything going wrong
Days full of laughter not having a care
Doing anything for fun or for a dare

Playing football all hours of the day
The hours simply disappeared out of the way
Always being part of the in crowd
Being boisterous shouting and screaming out loud

Then we would play cricket all summer long
Bruised arms and legs but doing nothing wrong
Bowling and batting as well as we could
The great sound of leather on wood

Next we would all hang around in a gang
Listening to favourite music we joined in and sang
Our numbers ranged from 4 up to 20
The banter we had was great and plenty

HERO

To say that I'm your hero that meant so much
That you say I'm your idol my heart was touched
I hope you can look up to me
I want you to be whatever you want to be

You can tell me all your hopes and fears
Share my laughter and cry my tears
All together we can pull through
As long as we are honest and true

Try your best that's all you can do
I can't ask any more from any of you
You bring so much joy into my life
To see you upset cuts like a knife

So talk to me ask whatever you want
I will always answer I won't say I can't
I will be there for you no matter when
You can call on me again and again

Look on me as your best friend
Whatever I have you can have or lend
I will share with you the lessons that I know
My love for you will always grow

NEIL

Picking a random radio station one out of the blue
A song comes on one that reminds me of you
Feelings of emptiness now that your gone
You left so early why did it go wrong

I suppose people say its one of those things
I remember your sister's voice when the phone
rings
The news she told me still haunts me today
That such a great guy has been taken away

So I will always remember you when I hear that
song
Always have that internal tear but not for too long
Then I will have a small smile on my face
The memory of you can never be replaced

To die so young just doesn't seem fair
Tears from everyone we showed we all cared
So here in my heart you will always remain
Earths great loss is heavens incredible gain

I hope you are there looking down on me
I'm sure you smile how bizarre my life can be
So when we meet up we will I think
I look forward to a joke and to a drink

Just remember how much I thought of you
Please show me a sign or give me a clue
Time will pass but not too long
Before I hear our favourite song

HOW WOULD I KNOW

How can I judge if I'm getting any better
Should I keep a diary or write it in a letter
Why has it happened to me how can it be
That I'm always drowning in a sea of uncertainty

Three years has passed and I'm none the wiser
How can that be does it surprise you
You can't just keep increasing the medication
The more I have just clouds the situation

It seems to get it right is a lottery
If one doesn't work try another one, two or three?
But what are the side effects and at what cost
Do I have to pay with years that are lost?

You say there's no cure you are only able to treat
the symptoms
But that's always playing catch up no clear
solutions
Should I wean myself off my medicine addiction?
Would I be better off not having that restriction?

STALLED

My life seems to be permanently on hold
I feel I've lost my grip I've lost my control
I'm scared of the future and what might be
Wondering if I will ever find the real me

Having more questions than answers is how it
seems
Feeling so isolated not part of the team
I suppose it's true that we're all unique
But do people judge me as some kind of freak

If I ask you to swap with me I wonder if you would
dare
Maybe then you would understand and you would
start to care
You would see what it's like in this living hell
Will I ever get better or start to feel well

Where I am today could well happen to you
It can creep up on you come out of the blue
How would you cope how would you feel
You would think it's a fantasy but boy is it real

Well mental illness isn't speaking about its taboo
It affects one in four people that's a fact its true
So let's bring it out in the open lets all make a
stand
Lay our cards on the table no more underhand

Perhaps in time the stigma will go

People's knowledge and education will begin to
grow
Then we would be more accepted in society
And this would be a better place for me to be

REALITY CHECK

Thinking of how I would like to be
A more fulfilled person richer a better me
Trying to leave my past behind
To do my small bit for all of mankind

I would like to change things and make them
better
Write things down and post myself a letter
To tell myself how I could change
Shake up my system start to re-arrange

Time to move on and set a new goal
Not to sell out to the devil but to save my soul
Try to feel that I'm born again
Maybe then I can release all my pain

My mind feels like it's going to explode
Mentally and physically I am on total overload
Time to relax a need to reflect
Try to feel very positive and not to reject

Into the future where will I be a year from now?
Will I have moved on and be able to look back at
how
To how I felt and the emotions I feel
I'm sure I will remember them they were oh so real

I suppose it's all a learning curve
Have I the bottle do I have the nerve
To carry out plans I have in my mind

To learn to be more gentle, understanding and kind

NEVER ENDING CIRCLE

Like a never ending circle where does it all start?
Can it be dissected looked into cut and torn apart?
Where did this illness begin will it ever end
Is it my own ghost or some long lost friend?

Try to make the most of the good days enjoy them
if I can
Live each day for that day is there some master
plan
To help me on the bad days to somehow pull me
through
Try to be more understanding is all I ask of you

Living in the present is what I need to do
Not raking over what might have been some kind
of hidden clue
Hopefully more happy times ahead and put the
past behind
Be more spontaneous more helpful and more kind

I don't need to be a sheep following the mass
Just want to be the best in my own special class
If I can teach to people then I also have to learn
To be a free spirit would that cause you concern

So if I'm to get off this life's merry go round
I have to try and do my best keep both feet on the
ground
Never to be frightened what lies ahead for me
Looking forward to what's in store in my life's
mystery

GUILTY

Why is it I feel so guilty when I've done nothing
wrong
When will I get better when will it be, how long
Am I hoping for something that's never going to be
Will I have to adjust my goals to find the real me

I don't seem to be getting any better not even a bit
I know it takes time but I'm so fed up with it
If I could change my life, have my destiny in my
own hands
Could I achieve my goals and carry out my plans

I would like you to be proud of me because I only
feel shame
To let it all wash over me there's no one to blame
I'm so tired being full of all your medication
Maybe I should start my own private revolution

You see the thoughts I have are so bizarre
Most of them seem to come from someone afar
Just to find peace of mind at any price
Being free from guilt and stigma would be nice

I hope I can look forward with no more looking
back
Then the wheels would start rolling down the right
track
Hoping for more fun and being happy every day
These feelings must never be forgot I hope and
pray

So I suppose the answers I need are all in my
head
Bit by bit I will start doing whatever I have said
I hope there's time to do everything that I wish
Then I will be in a big river being the big fish

LOW

Depression creeps up on me I don't even know
What are the warning signs they don't seem to
show
The feeling of being so depressed and down
It's hard to smile and easy to frown

Some days I don't want to get out of my bed
Lying there trying to clear my head
But the fuzziness is always there
No more spontaneous things I have to prepare

Take the medicine day after day
But does it work well who am I to say
They say it takes time to work
Well if that's true
Can I speed up the process and stop feeling so
blue

In the future not knowing what's next for me
Leaves me drowning in this mental uncertainty
How can I stop myself from going under
Can I stop the storm the lightening and the
thunder

When I feel that things can't get any worse
They do, is this some kind of sick curse
Is there some magic that can break the spell
To get me back to normal to start feeling well

Then I can go back to living my life

Leave the past behind leave all the strife
Being able to be where I want to be
Then I would be happy playing simple me

UNFAIR

Why is it that I feel that life is so unfair
I'm just glad I've got you and that you all care
Why is it that I'm not getting or feeling any better
I've stuck to all the rules right down to the last
letter

For three years we have had this burden around
our necks
How do we get rid of it clear the decks
Life's so unfair at times and I don't know why
I've recently asked myself why me it always
makes me cry

Only you know the pain that we've been through
Our love is the purest so honest and true
Without you I've nothing to fight on for
We've got that small ray of light shining through
the door

We have to be patient it just takes time
But time moves on and I feel like I've done some
crime
To be like this rips me straight through the heart
Even though we are not together we will never be
apart

ALONE

It hurts so much that we are once again apart
It leaves me with a big gap a hole in my heart
Just being near you makes me feel so much better
It's so hard for me to write it down in a love letter

I'm determined to get it right so that we can move on
Without you all I don't feel a complete person
Every minute that I'm away from you all
Makes me feel small where once I was tall

Hopefully we won't be apart for too long
Maybe you remember me from words in a song
Just never forget me just keep me in mind
My love for you all is oh so clear and will never be blind

You're my reason to keep battling and fighting
I can't wait for the moment when we are reuniting
I will always love you for ever and a day
No matter what obstacles come up in our way?
I'm so proud of the way that you all cope
So I'm never going to give up because there's always hope

REPETITIVE FEELING

Why do I have this repetitive feeling?
That I can't see the light nothing I'm seeing
The tunnel ahead always seems so dark
No glimmer of hope not even a spark

Time stands still for no man I know its true
But me getting better is now so long overdue
If I knew that things would soon turn around
I would be able to stop screaming without any
sound

I feel I'm always being punished when I've done
nothing wrong
Feeling isolated having the internal torture for so
long
Is it only me that can sort this all out
Tell me why I'm like this what's it all about

Thoughts in my head they seem so bizarre
I'm always standing still but I feel I've travelled so
far
I will never give up because then I've lost
But boy am I paying well over the cost

TINA

You must feel so trapped in a world of your own
Not letting anyone in are you happy all alone
Can you reveal what's going on in your mind?
You've got perfect vision but have still ended up
blind

Has your medication locked away all your desire
Your body's on auto pilot but do you require
Peace of mind a chance to be able and free
To fight your own demons and all that you see

How do you break the vicious cycle that goes
round?
Do you have plans to get your feet back on the
ground?
Who's helping you whose fighting your cause
Or are you happy with your life permanently set on
pause

If you don't help yourself then hell who will
Your batteries are on empty you're running to a
stand still
Hours turn to days to weeks even to years
This isn't a trip saying wish you were here

HUMAN ZOO

How can it be you spent over a year of your life
Trapped in a system that's given you trouble and
strife
Caught up in a world that's so small and intense
To break out of the system you've created has to
be your intent

I can hardly imagine how it must feel for you
Caged up in an institution like a human zoo
You must have seen so many people come and
go
But you never seem angry or let your feelings
show

So you say your moving on to pastures new
But this place will always be a big part of you
I am pleased to have met you if only for a while
No matter what you've gone through you still
manage to smile

So I wish you luck as you go on your way
I will spare a little thought for you each and every
day
I hope they can help you and you start to feel
good
Then you will get the life you want like everyone
should

W G and N

I miss the three of you so very much
To have you near to me, to feel, to touch
It hurts it feels like I've let you down
It's so unfair on you that I'm not around

For most of the last three years it's been like this
If things could be made right with a magic wish
I will promise I will fight to make sure I'm better
You can remind me of this and show me this letter

The way you handle things makes me so proud
To do things together is what we should be
allowed
To be able to leave all bad things in the past
To do what we want together and to have a laugh

With all of you helping I will soon get there
The love and affection you give me shows you
care
In the future I promise that things will be great
I will be your dad your bestest loyal mate
So hold me to these words and they will come true
I love you so much I love all of you

(God Bless)

HOW THINGS SHOULD BE

When I'm better how things should be
A new born again person but deep down still me
Enjoying normal things without having a care
Just nice real dreams and not a constant
nightmare

No more being frightened and being scared
They say for me to win then I have to dare
To take chances live life on the edge of a knife
Try not to be cut but to get on with my life

Will I be able to be free of all this medication?
So I can think clear without any chemical sedation
To have my emotions under my own control
Not feeling like I'm always in a public goldfish bowl

So let's hope that it doesn't take too long
To put right everything that has gone wrong
Then I wouldn't feel so much out of place
The smile you see would be real on my face

SPINNING HEAD

Back to where I know like the back of my hand
Different people nothing that I would have planned
This is the place I need to be right here and now
Use it for what it is and get through somehow

I have to go through the pain barrier and reach the
other side
Put up with the rough and tumble and swallow all
my pride
I will try not to panic I must be strong and brave
Tired of this chemical imbalance I feel such a
slave

I need things to change so that I can start to live
There is so much I have on offer so much for me
to give
The learning curve just seems to take so long
For every two rights I seem to have three wrongs

The times right to feel like I'm born again
Get through this mental torture feel the pain
At the end of the tunnel there must be a light
Well I'm going to search for it not give up the fight

So to take control be a man once more
And stand up right make it through my life's door
To enter into a much happier place
And lose the frown and have a smile on my face

JANE

When I saw you tonight I saw the pain in your face
Words can't express the unpleasantness and bad taste
I felt that in some way that I had let you down
I know how much hurt you feel when I'm not around

The day we met is now so long ago
I loved you so much so soon and that love still grows
Beyond anything that I thought I could ever feel
You're loved by me so much it sometimes seems so surreal

Without you I would be no one nothing a man all alone
I would be like some stray dog looking for his lost bone
I sit here now shedding a tear how much you care
It's at a time like this when life seems so unfair

I will sleep tonight and dream of my love for you
Hopefully one day all our dreams will come true
Then we will have the time of our lives
I want to make you the happiest wife
So you can be proud of me for things that I've done
The battles nearly over just the war to be won

Jane I love you with all of my heart

WHO ARE YOU

Who are you I can see where you're from
Walking around like you own the place I was that
one
The trouble is your so high you just wait for the
crash
The feelings that you have now I promise they
won't last

I would give you advice but would you listen to me
I see your the person that I used to be
But when you fall who will you run to
You will be isolated alone out there just you

So enjoy the feeling of being so elated
With your massive ego which will soon become
deflated
Then the real test for you will start to begin
You will have to fight the demons you have from
within

So you can live in a fantasy world if that's where
you are
Living in your own bubble your very own super
star
But no one wants to see your one man side show
Your moving way too fast everyone else is so slow

So I think I can see where you are going to be
On the slippery slope uncertain of your sanity
It's a one way ticket out into the unknown

But there's a lot of me in you, you will never be alone

FRUSTRATION

I'm so frustrated not knowing where to turn
I don't feel any the wiser but can I still learn
Wishing for a change of life's fortune
Praying it's not too long to see a change soon

How long will it take if anyone knew?
Then I could look ahead no more stuck in glue
Why is it I feel permanently on hold?
It feels like my soul has been sold

I suppose I'm hoping for some kind of guarantee
That I'm not damaged goods for everyone to see
I try to put up a barrier not let it show
Does that help anyone I suppose the answers no

If anyone can show me the way to survive
So it makes me feel that I'm ok and I'm still alive
Then I will follow that path without looking back
Hoping that I will never fall off my destiny's track

ROOM 101

What five things do I detest and want to throw
away
What could I put in my room never again to see
the light of day?
Things that I would be a lot better off without
Five things to get rid of I'm certain there's no
doubt

First thing to put into the room is the stigma
around mental health
No more a taboo subject or something to leave on
a shelf
Ridding everyone of their ignorance there's really
no excuse
Having more compassion towards our illness
rather than verbal abuse

Second to go in for everyone to be free from
poverty
The world's wealth to be shared equally put
poverty to history
Why should a few have so much more than they
need?
Divide it between everyone eliminate all greed

Third item I would throw racism straight in the bin
How can you judge someone just by the colour of
their skin?
Or because they look or speak differently to you

Don't stereotype the mass of a race for the sake of
an extreme few

Fourth thing to go would be an end to all the
world's terrorists
Fighting against their own people's needs fighting
against their wish
Putting so many people in fear each and every
day
Not caring about innocent people they destroy
whilst getting their way

Fifth and final thing to get rid of to end all of the
world wars
Each and everyone being friendly to each other no
more settling old scores
Then everyone would be more relaxed happy and
at ease
All over the world a white flag flying the start of
world peace

2005 THE YEAR GONE

As the end of the year approaches fast
Reflect on the 12 months that have past
At the start I had so much hope
I had to draw on resources to simply cope

When I thought things couldn't get worse they did
And for so long I managed to keep all the signs
well hid
But my depression deepened I had to tell
Things had to get worse for me to get well

To isolate myself for such a long time
Trying to clear out rubbish from my mind
Having to dig deep just to stay in control
To stop me entering another black hole

I suppose the year was a learning curve
To see if I could win and hold my nerve
I didn't consider it a contest I could lose
Just to look at my options and be free to choose.

So as the year ends how do things look?
Another end of a chapter in my life's book
I'm still here standing after taking more blows
Watch this space let's see how it goes

THE YEAR END

The end of the year a time to reflect and look back
Try to think of the things I have rather than the
things I lack
It's been a year to forget probably the worst I have
ever had
But I have made it through somehow so I should
be glad

If someone had told me 12 months ago how it
would be
So much stress and depression bearing down on
me
When things got worse I went further down
Having to dig so deep I'm just glad you've been
around

I sometimes forget the effect this condition has on
you
You live everyday along with it you always pull
through
I'm proud of the way you manage to stay so strong
Against all the bad times we've had when things
have gone wrong

Thinking back on the year it seems to have gone
in a flash
Somehow managing to escape from another life's
car crash
Hopefully now things can move onwards and
upwards

Try not to look back too much, concentrate on moving forwards

I will never forget the friend's, family that we've lost this year
They all hold a special place in my heart of that I'm sincere
I'll try not to be sad when I remember any of you
Remembering the good and happy times and try not to rue
If things had been different well that's a big word IF
Things are how they are for a reason even if that's against my wish

SAD

Feeling sad is an emotion I know so well
Don't ask me how I feel I'm sure you can tell
Why do I feel so sad most of the time?
Imprisoned by my mental illness is that a crime?

Feeling empty feeling I've run out of gas
I've had this emotion for so long when will it pass
When I motivate myself and do things I enjoy
I feel better for a short while then I go coy

The sadness seems permanently etched on my
face
A smile appears but it's always out of place
Can I ever feel well and be at ease
To be carefree and be able to do as I please

I know everyone feels sad but me more than most
It haunts and follows me around my holy ghost
The hope I have is one day my sadness will go
Then my happy and good emotions will be allowed
to show

SCARED (2)

Scared of the future scared of the past
Scared of the feelings that always seem to last
Terrified of the moment I find myself in
Waiting for a brand new moment to begin

Scared that the time just seems to fly by
Not any great improvement I ask myself why
That even though I try as hard as I can
Nothing seems to work no matter how I plan

So is being scared going to always be with me
Or can I toss it away and start to feel free
No more panicky feeling oh how I wish
How good life could be if it was like this

Finally being able to go forward and move on
To feel that the bad memories are finally gone
But a start would be just enough to be less scared
So I can get myself ready so I know that I'm
prepared

LOWER THAN ROCK BOTTOM

Why is it when I've reached rock bottom I go lower
Why is it that medication is not working time goes
slower
I'm told it takes time but how long will that be
Can I be reborn again become the real me

The dreams I have are not too much to ask
Just simple things not a difficult task
But I'm doing everything by the book
So why does it feel I've run out of luck

Frustration sets in feelings of deep despair
I wonder who understands who really cares
If I could pull myself together that's what I would
do
A miracle cure would be so great it's so long
overdue

Dark thoughts are constantly spinning around in
my head
Sometimes it feels like I'm living a life that's dead
Things people take for granted it doesn't seem fair
I have to dig deeper each day being awake in this
nightmare

But whatever happens I will never give up hope
Having faith strength and courage is how I cope
When I'm desperate and banging my head against
the wall
Please be there for me when I shout and call

It feels like I've been given a life sentence
Not being able to make a decision always sat on the fence
Please help me move forward in the right direction
To somehow get me by this mental illness situation

I WISH

I wish that I was well and no longer ill
To feel that I'm not always climbing up this mental
hill
Never knowing how I'm going to be
Struggling and soul searching to find the real me

I wish to feel the same as the majority
To be able to appreciate the feeling of normality
Never ever going forever up and down
Feeling level with both feet firmly on the ground

I wish I could put a smile upon your face
Not to be prejudged or to feel that I'm out of place
To go through life without a worry or a care
Being able to be more adventurous prepared to
take a dare

I wish that I was like the me that you used to know
But so many things have changed and that was
long ago
So I have to accept and do all that I can
To be a better person to become a better man

So if I depend solely on wishes and if they don't
come true
I would feel let down and end up feeling blue
So hopefully in my own hands will be my own
destiny
To open up life's door and let me start a new
journey

KNOWING ME

Am I a better person than I used to be
Can I break free from my own history?
I know I cannot change what's gone on before
But I can fight the disease try and find a cure

I'm so glad that your there for me
The day we met must have been destiny
Without you I would be left all alone
Nothing to live for a future unknown

You know me better than I know myself
You stopped me from being left on the shelf
One day I hope to be able to make you feel so proud
So that you can stand up and shout out loud

That I've achieved what I set out to do
But these are things I can only do if I have you
Your support means the world to me
It's obvious that we were meant to be

The hardest battle has to be fought
We will draw on lessons that we've been taught
I know we will get there one way or another
Because the main thing is that we've got each other

You and I together will stand side by side
Hearts entwined we won't have to hide
We will face the world together head on
You will always be my number one

MR NOBODY

You think you know someone how they appear
But opinions can change all is not that clear
Your not the person I thought I knew
Are you ill or is what I'm seeing the real you
If you've a problem with me please let me know
You've let down your guard the cracks do show

You walk around like you own the place
But the way you talk to people is a disgrace
You moan about people but your the biggest
moaner of all
One day you will get what you deserve a great big
fall
If your as clever and as smart as you think
Why when you try to walk on water is it you
always sink

The plans you have change each and every day
But I'm smarter than you and remember what you
say
One day you slag someone off the next their great
I'm always polite to you but don't call me mate
The illness you have is the same as mine
But I can behave I know how to tow the line

In a week you state that you will be free
But don't build your hopes up there's no guarantee
What you want is not always what you get
You've told me things that I'm never going to
forget

Everyone's glad when you've passed by
Perhaps open your eyes and ask yourself why

I might be wrong in my opinion of you
So if I am then an apology is due
But I'm sure I've seen the real man
If you can be called a man then anyone can
So now I've said my peace I will leave you in
peace
My chastation of you will now cease

CONCERT

We set off early gave ourselves plenty of time
The weather was windy but with some sunshine
We arrived within an hour which was great
We parked close by we had hours to wait

Found the stadium ok but had to walk miles
around
Had to find the correct entrance to the football
ground
Once inside we were directed to our seats
Several thousand people already there feeling the
heat

After a few hours the first band on stage
They were quite good a half hour set they played
After a short break the next act appeared
Everyone in the mood a party atmosphere
An hour set that went down really great
The crowd was up to 25,000 there were some that
were late

A short break before the main event
People buying t-shirts programmes money well
spent
You walked on stage the place erupted
A 5 minute ovation that wasn't interrupted

Straight into your first song we all danced away
The stands were bouncing hit after hit you played
Everyone was singing dancing cheering too

The pure admiration directed towards you

Time passed more than 2 hours had gone
A brilliant time had been had by everyone
Back on for a final curtain call
A standing ovation again by each and all
A brilliant time a wonderful day
Lots of great memories to take away

A TRUE FRIEND

I would like to write my own special tribute to you
I think we clicked from day one you're a friend
that's true
You know that I don't bullshit what I say is meant
You're a person I admire to me a real gent

I know how hard life's been this last 18 months for
you
But you've got a strong character that will see you
through
Don't be too hard on yourself because your ill
don't feel shame
What happened to you wasn't your fault you know
you're not to blame

I have met many people along my mental health
journey
But you're the one who's made the biggest
impression on me
You've always took time out to ask and see how I
am
In my eyes that makes you a special person a
special kind of man

So I hope in some way we bonded and we can
stay friends
Let's keep in touch see each other so our
friendship never ends
If ever you need to chat to meet up just keep in
touch

I would like to stay mates forever I would like that very much

A TRUE ANGEL

Sometimes you meet up with someone you
connect straight away
Their always there for you listening to what you
have to say
They don't judge you they just show that they care
You can feel very vulnerable laid out naked and
bare

But you always seem to know the right things to
say
Words of encouragement that gets me through
each day
I don't think it's a skill that's taught more a natural
gift
When I'm at my lowest low you manage to give
me a lift

When I can't see a future and I am always feeling
down
You say how well I'm doing and that I can turn
things around
It's so hard to treat an illness one that's in one's
mind
But by being understanding and caring and by just
being kind

You go the extra mile I know how much you care
I'm so lucky to have you as my angel one who's
always there
I've been very lucky that you've been there for me

To help me get to the place I really want to be
So I thank you with all my heart and I wish you
well
You deserve a medal for what you do my special
angel

ALL ABOUT ME

All about me a story to tell
From a daily heaven to a living hell
How to begin oh where do I start
I'll tell it how it is straight from the heart

Well I was born Derbyshire bred
I will take you on a tour inside my head
I will try to be honest with the good and bad
Lots of things are happy many are sad

I had a good childhood the third child of four
Two brothers and one sister who could want more
A mum called Betty and a dad called Ray
Who looked after me each and every day

At school I was the one who acted the clown
Always told off and banned from the playground
I should have tried harder and could have done
much better
But all my parents got were warning letters

So all throughout school my life was fun
Nothing to worry about no need to run
No one had foreseen what lay ahead
The unwelcome demons were growing in my head

Left school with average grades oh what a shame
It was all my fault no one else was to blame
My dad got me a job as a trainee
At British Railway an apprenticeship for me

Work was ok we all had a laugh
Working away we all acted daft
College was hard real graft to do
But I was really happy not at all blue

But then at 19 life was so cruel
I had done nothing wrong I had played by the
rules
Paranoid panicky no sleep as well
My first experience of living in hell

The thoughts I had are still clear today
But I will spare you from them I will lock them
away
You wouldn't have liked what was inside my head
Like an unfinished book there are lots more to be
read

There are lots more to tell you so much more to
come
Another 20 years of shear hell plus lots of fun
But I will stop for now I will leave the rest
Until another day when I will tell my quest

WISHES

Wishes are things that we all have
To take them seriously or treat as a laugh
We all hope that they can come true
I will open up some of my secrets and share a few

I wish that people were made more aware
Not to prejudge but to love and care
To be more compassionate and understanding
Not to be scared of me crash landing

I wish that people's knowledge would flourish and
grow
They wouldn't make excuses turn their backs on
me and go
If they would treat me as an equal and just the
same
I would be able to share my thoughts not have to
hide in shame

I wish that people would listen to me
Hear what I say be able to hear my plea
Instead most people just seem to walk away
But a mental illness could happen to you one day

So if I have a final wish one hope for you
If ever you are down or just feeling blue
In me you have someone who really cares
Just call on me and I will be there

WISH

A wish is a dream that I've never had
It's something to reach out for when things are bad
It's a way of hoping and dreaming how things could be
All thrown together reality and fantasy

So many times I've forgot my dreams
If I only knew the plots knew the schemes
Memories start to fade but scars always remain
To rise back up to the surface to feel I'm born again

I wish that there's no more pain
I wish that there's no hidden shame
I dream of how my future will be
On forever in a heavenly eternity

My wishes for you are simple and pure
To have them all come true and for so much more
To have the freedom to feel released
With no more worries then I would be pleased

So dream of happiness because it will come
Dream of being positive not being over run
Live life to the full the burden of cares
Let life be a wonderful dream and not a nightmare

MAX

For a few days I thought I was losing you
My world fell apart I was oh so blue
You've been there for me for 3 years now
You've shared my pain we've got through
somehow

Without you my life would be so empty
The love you give me is unconditional and plenty
I could see the hurt it was in your eyes
But you're a fighter like me that's no surprise

So you seem to be getting better lets hope
To be without you would be so hard to cope
The journey for you well how will it end?
You're my one and only, a man's best friend

So we've been through the thick and the thin
As one story stops another begins
It's true you're loved with all my heart
Let's pray for the future we're never apart

2006

Before we've even finished singing auld langs ine
Thoughts go swirling around inside my mind
Of the year that's gone and thank god it has
A year to forget and leave well in the past

A new year a new start filled with new hope to
A year to find answers do I search for a clue
To find the person I so long want to be
The feeling of being born again washes over me

No longer to feel scared of what's in my head
Motivating myself to get up and out of bed
Try as hard as I can to stay focused and strong
To get back to a place where I know I belong

I know things have moved on and I feel so left
behind
Why is this condition of mine so cruel and unkind?
I know in some ways that I've become a new man
But I have no real control of who I really am

One thing I've learnt is that I have to be honest
Even when I'm at my worst I must try my best
To get through each and every day no matter what
Not to get upset of memories of things I have
forgot

So to take one day at a time is how it's going to be
Not running before I can walk to find my true
destiny
Given time I will learn from all my mistakes

And try to have a great year whatever it may take

SMALL STEPS

Lying in bed trying to sleep
Things spinning around secrets to keep
Could I tell could I explain
Will my life ever be the same

Some thoughts normal some are strange
Try to sort them out try to re-arrange
It's hard to explain the internal screaming
The pains still there even when I'm dreaming

So I will always be honest open and true
Try not to panic if one day I'm blue
Knowing the pain won't always last
Not frightened by the ghost of my past

Take small steps day by day
Take the punches on the chin or dodge out the way
I'm sure one day things will be fine
It's just that small question of time

So in the future how will it be
When I look in the mirror whose reflection will I see?
Will it be me slowly sinking and drowning
Or standing proud confident no more frowning

What will happen tomorrow well no one knows
But I want to stay focused and deal with the blows
And if I can remain positive and strong

Then a wonderful journey I will have come join along

MY EMOTIONS

Things inside my mind are never very clear
All mixed up with hopes and dreams but shrouded
with fear
If I opened up my mind then you could take a look
There's so much going on in there I ought to write
a book

My mind is sometimes normal whatever normal is
It sometimes races oh so fast time goes by at a
whiz
So when my mind is racing it's so hard for me to
explain
Excitement, fear, panic, ecstasy and pain

Smiling, joking, loving everyone laughter all
around
Then crying tears of real pain for no reason that
can be found
One minute on the highest high and then the
lowest low
Just when things seem to be going good they
simply vanish and go

So losing the plot isn't easy I got tossed and
hurled
I'm telling you some of my very own Wayne's
world
It's a unique journey one I've gone alone

39 years and counting don't condemn or condone

DON'T PUSH ME

Don't push me too far I might just explode
I will only take so much you may overload
Then you will see the other side of me
What about the consequences what will be will be

Well you know I'm a lot stronger than you
I can play mind games and no one would have a
clue
So this is a promise and not a threat
Just leave me alone or else you will regret

Don't hide behind mental illness to say what you
want
I could easily do that but my morals say I can't
Your not the only one who can upset and confuse
I will let you decide how it will be you can choose

Well you know that I'm just as ill that's why I'm
here
So give me some space don't come any nearer
Perhaps I've got more insight into my illness
But I'm not going to share it with you because it's
my business

HIGH

Let me try and explain to you how my illness is
It's not a pretty story but it goes like this
For no apparent reason I can go really high
To feel real ecstasy to feel way up in the sky

When I feel like this it's brilliant to start
But it can't carry on this feeling tears me apart
If only I could stay at a level that's nice
I wouldn't ask for anything more that would suffice

To feel super confident not to have a care
Never having any worries no need to prepare
Being able to face whatever comes my way
Living life to the max each and every day

From the outside you say there's nothing wrong
That I shouldn't be ill for this long
You tell me to be strong and brave
You're scared of the way I sometimes behave

People who don't know me wouldn't know
What's wrong with me because it doesn't show
They say there's nothing wrong with you and just
to move on
But that's far easier said than to be done

So if I could bottle the high and give some to you
Then you would feel born again and brand new
If it could be given to all the human race
Then this world would be a much better place

LET ME BE UNDERSTOOD

I try to stay positive take it day by day
Set small goals and targets get help along the way
And if things go wrong as they sometimes can
Don't be hard on myself I've got another plan

Always try to be honest open and true
Try not to beat myself up when I feel blue
I have to stay focused be helpful and kind
Try and lead from the front not be left behind

So I've told you some of my ups and downs
There's lots of secrets to be found
One day I would like to share it all
But not quite yet I'm scared I'll fall

So here's to the future whatever will be
Things are starting to become clear for me
Hopefully no more hurt and only good
Then I would be fulfilled and understood

STOOD STILL

How can I move on when I'm always standing still
Could I find a way to climb an endless hill
What it takes is a small step at a time
But I cannot see those steps when the feet are
mine

I'm told by everyone not to panic or to worry
But that's easier said than done I'm always saying
sorry
I feel that I have let so many people down
My illness just seems to go around and around

I cannot change my past even if I tried
What's gone has gone and cannot be denied
So I will have to be the best I can each and every
day
Try to get over any obstacles that get in my way

It's like climbing out of a very deep hole
You get so far out but can never reach your goal
So many small lifts but never quite enough
God no one tells you bipolar is so tough

<u>DREAMS</u>

Dreams can come true if you try hard
Pictures in the mind like some greeting card
Paradise a place on earth for all to see
A future of happiness for you and me

Not more bad luck no more mirrors to break
A chilled out future life's one big birthday cake
A piece for each and everyone to share
Living in the present without a care

PRE-DIAGNOSE

Which way to go which way to turn
To young to forget to old to learn
No place to return to, too much hurt pride
Everywhere to run to but nowhere to hide

All twisted up inside shrieks of pain
Could we re-track, retrace start to regain
What that was once taken for granted without
thought
Not learnt in a classroom but must be self-taught

The one to bear the burden, hurt and shame
Tears for dice it's the crying game
While other's go by not towing the line
What's theirs is ours but yours is not mine

To grow up with fear of noises in the night
To hold inside the internal fright
Not knowing who to turn to
You don't always get what's supposedly due

WHAT CHOICE

What choice should I make for the best
Do I count this as the biggest test
Is there a plan A or B for me
I feel I'm drowning in uncertainty

Asking for help I know the need
Conflicting stories I just won't heed
The hardest decision I had to make
If only life was to give and not to take

I'm living with a spinning head
Must fight the fight and relax in bed
If I could stop the spinning for just an hour
Then I might regain some of my power

SILENCE

Emptiness without a noise
Mind games without the toys
Could this be a never ending story
Winning wars without the glory

Open up talk and tell
Break the black shrouded spell
Time moves on fast and slow
Speeding thoughts will they ever go

Stay positive, unwind get better
Write myself an honest get well letter
Love will pull me through again
And to the past these thoughts will remain

FAULTS

Faults that lie in everyone
Can't be perfect all things can't be done
All in good time we will find the truth
But can it be clear do we know the truth

How to go right or wrong
The path is short but the road so long
If it was easy it would be done
The battles lost but the war could be won

Every breath we take is fresh and new
The sky can be grey but when it's blue
It lifts us up to a higher high
We know there's something that will see us by

WE DESERVE

We deserve what we get but that's so cruel
Nobody should have the right to set the rules
To be with each other and all be the same
No rules need to be broken just fun and games

To live without fear to live without fright
To be at the end of the tunnel where there is light
That's a place I so want to be
I will be there one day I promise you see

To be the best I can I must try
Don't be afraid if I start to cry
Will get back where we all belong
Happy smiles, laughter and songs

POWER STRUGGLE

To see the power struggle is a farce
Half the people here should get off their arse
They seem to be pulling some kind of con
With their nasty ways until their deeds are done

Watch my back at all times
Look out for those danger signs
Talk to the staff get quick help
Don't hold it all in my head it's going to pulp

To be well to go in a week or two
But if it's longer that's something I'll have to do
Don't need to take risks or to take dares
All the help and support is always there

GET TO HIM

Get to him somehow but don't know
Try not to let the anger and the feelings show
Time to show some real true grit
But only be prepared to take so much shit

I can start to play the mind games
Make him feel humiliated and ashamed
Take more steps one by one
Take away his credit till it's all gone

Teach him a lesson he'll never forget
Reel him in like a fish into a net
Speed up things at the double
Keep my nose clean but get him in trouble

CHALK AND CHEESE

A friendly smile and being polite
A nice good morning and a nice good night
Time to relax and to be at ease
But then you change like chalk and cheese

Work in the system just for fun
Pulling the wool over their eyes your one big con
Some are real some are fake
Turn your back and the thieves will take

So the warning that I give to you
Is to be honest, real and be true
If your not then you will be caught
Something to think about, food for thought

BAGPUSS

Bitter and twisted that's what you are
Acting like your some kind of superstar
A face like shit a frown as well
Really ill ha not a cat in hell

Everyone hates the sound of your voice
We leave the room by choice
If the world's against you no one cares
Leave everyone alone real problems are shared

You blame everyone except for yourself
But like a book gathering dust on the shelf
So you don't like me, so what
I don't listen to you, not one jot

SHE

She talked about us as if she didn't care
She looked straight through us as if we weren't there
We are all human beings but she called us "them"
Treated us like we were in a pig pen

No manners at all, well not to us
We were being treated like we were second class
One day it could be her sat in that chair
Would she complain about her level of care

This is not fiction this is true
So much to change but by so few
Manic depression oh what is that
Well don't treat us all like we're all twats

MY BRAVE FACE

To hold it all in not to let is show
Afraid what might happen if I let it go
Am I strong enough to come through this
Walk the tight rope and take the risk

The smile covers the pain inside
No self esteem not one bit of pride
Is this going to happen again and again
Like a caged lion for ever stuck in a den

I have the will to beat and overcome
Put things right complete the total sum
If questions are asked and never denied
Then trouble and peace will always be side by
side

DESERTED

I feel like a big part of me has been ripped away
Not being in control not knowing what to say
It's so hard to look to the future when my past has
gone
My life seems so cruelly finished before it has
begun

The tears I've cried and cried will they ever stop
My eyes stinging so sore can I ever make it back
to the top
I suppose deep down I knew it would come to this
But it doesn't make it easier it's something I'm
going to miss

You see I had a dream and a vision of how things
would be
Now that's been ripped away and taken from me
I hear you say it might be a blessing in disguise
Only time will tell let's hope there's a good
surprise

So at the moment I just feel gutted and deserted
When I needed help most, well did I deserve this
I suppose I'm hoping for answers that no one
knows
But it's hurting me and the pain and strain shows

HISTORY REPEATS ITSELF

Here we go again as history repeats itself
Abandoned on my own feeling left upon the shelf
People say don't worry but that's easier said than
done
Has my life been prematurely ended or as a new
me begun

Even when something is half expected there's still
a half that's not
I will try my hardest to get through this I will give it
my best shot
I know that things in time go forward and that
things move on
But I feel so scared and frightened I'm the isolated
one

I suppose if I'm honest I've known I won't go back
With no confidence to call on struggling with panic
attacks
But still I'm left with such a bad taste in my mouth
I need my mood to head up north not stuck in the
Deep South

So once the dust has settled there are things I
won't forget
I know that I can bounce back I'm not going to be
finished yet
So I will be left with memories way more good
than bad

And I will try to think of positive things be happy and not sad

BLESSING IN DISGUISE

I thank you for all your words and advice you have
given me
I'm so glad I've real friends that say your futures
bright you'll see
I've cried so many tears I guess that's no surprise
You tell me that this will all end up being a
blessing in disguise

I know my mind just needs a rest time for it to
mend
To be free from this illness, which is my demon
and my friend
To take my brain away to a place where it can rest
Being able to recharge myself so I can be the best

Then to a time where I can move on never looking
back
To newer and better things in perfect condition no
more cracks
Walking around happy and content a smile upon
my face
No more panicky feelings no more falling from
grace

So here's to a positive future one where I belong
Doing what is good for me with nothing going
wrong
Drawing on all my experience helping others on
their way
Living life to the maximum forever and a day

ABANDONED

Abandoned is a word to describe the way that I feel
Something which started as a bad thought has turned out to be real
I know the reasons for your decision but it still hurts like hell
You say it will be a good thing well only time will tell

Don't tell me that you understand I don't see how you can
You have taken away my dignity left me a broken man
Trying to pick myself up but still reeling from the blows
You say that it will help me well let's see how it goes

8 years may not seem too long but it's a big part of my life
But that's about to be severed cut off by a knife
No longer a target or maybe a burden, well we will see
The path I have to follow to reach my destiny

I know deep down you have been very good to me
You could have left me shipwrecked stranded at sea
So really I must thank you with all of my heart
I'm just so very sorry that now we have to part

BLUES

If you understand what I'm saying then your the same as me
Some would say it is fate some kind of destiny
I never asked to be ill because no one would ever choose
This dark and empty vacuum is what I call my blues

I stuck to my medication but where has that got me
So tired and confused full of uncertainty
Can a cure for me be found in a certain pill
Or do they do me no good at all apart from keeping me feeling ill

I take pills to lift me up to stay stable stop me going high
But do any of them work at all I often ask myself why
Perhaps what is needed is for the stigma to be gone
And this internal shame I feel will start to be undone

So if you see me crying hanging my head feeling low
Just offer me a glimmer of hope a smile may even show
I will take my time step by step climbing one's not two's

Then you will know that I'm on my way back to hell with the blues

BLANK EXPRESSION

Why do you have a blank expression on your face
Do you think that a smile will be out of place
I know that look you give I've seen it many times
before
But I don't see any change in you when you go out
the door

I respect your point of view but I don't have to
agree
You see we're all unique even if your illness is the
same as me
Do I know myself better than you know you
I can admit when something's wrong but you don't
have a clue

So you think your more advanced further down the
line
But I can see your pitfalls because I'm over mine
So if you come back down to earth with one
almighty bang
Join back up with us become part of our gang

Our club is not exclusive new members do feel
free
To join our own special place it's sometimes
heavenly
Be prepared for anything because what happens
well who knows
It's one long rollercoaster journey one almighty
variety show

PANIC

The fear of panic seems to always be there
It's something I can't control it's just so unfair
Even if I can forget about it soon comes back and returns
I can't put into practice lessons that I've learned

I feel that everyone can see the panic in me
It's got a grip I can't escape please let me be free
My hearts beating so fast it's about to explode
My brain can't switch off its so full, complete overload

I can feel the sweat coming from each and every pore
Pumping out of me dripping onto the floor
I wish the ground could open up and just take me away
What I would do to be panic free for just a single day

Will there be a time in the future when the panic has gone
To have some confidence to be able to move on
Then I can be the person that I so long to be
Fulfil all my wishes and dreams with no more uncertainty

CONFUSED

So many thoughts rushing through my head
Thinking what might be after the things you've
said
I suppose I should feel happy but I don't so why
Do I feel like I'm standing still as time goes flying
by

You see things seem just too good to be true
Which usually means they are, so please give me
a clue
Of which pathway to take because I'm so
confused
I've had so much taken from me my mind battered
and bruised

Am I making things more complex than they need
to be
It's just the way that I am it's what makes me
My life always seems to be waiting for someone's
decision
So many vague notions I really need some
precision

Just to feel like things are going my way
To give me a little piece of mind just a little each
day
A chance for the mist to clear from my mind
Surely my life hasn't always got to be cruel to be
kind

ONE YEAR ON

It's one year on since you had to leave
So much has happened in that time it's hard to
believe
Not one day goes by without memories of you
Thinking of the fun you gave in the things that I do

It's seemed so sudden how you had to go
But my love for you goes on and still grows
I'm sure your happy now free from any pain
I'm certain we will be together and meet up again

I hope the time you had with us was time you
enjoyed
Was there more we could have done if so I'd be
so annoyed
Your there forever a place in my heart
Even though we are separated we will never be
apart

The emotions I have today are both happy and
sad
I will remember the good times and forget the bad
So your still there with me even though your gone
Your loved more than ever after one year on

PANICKY

Panic is a feeling I know so very well
I feel it creeping up on me I just know I can tell
I can feel my heart racing missing a beat
Even when it's very cold I start to sweat and feel
the heat

If I could run away and escape then I would
Can I learn to stop them well I wish I could
I feel the sweat pore out of me panic is setting in
I get so far then I fall again I have to begin

I slow my breathing down, deep breaths and relax
If only that would work for me but it doesn't that's
a fact
Panic has got a hold of me it always seems to win
I hear you say you can't tell but I know because
it's within

I suppose I have to learn to cope and get on with
my life
But if feels like I'm walking permanently on the
edge of a knife
So afraid of panic I just wish that it would go
Then I could move on the real me would show

BLACK

You asked me to describe the way that I feel
It's hard to explain it's sometimes quite surreal
I guess if I could express it as a colour rather than
a mood
Or a feeling of being starved left without any food

The colour I would have to pick would have to be
black
Because black covers everything and papers over
the cracks
Black is so dark and deep not a single hint of light
Internally I'm black and blue bruised from a life
long fight

You say that you can't feel black all of the time
Does that mean if I sometimes laugh or smile I've
committed a crime
I wish there was a rainbow out there waiting for
me
But with no flicker of light I'm left in total
uncertainty

I hear you say that this is a faze and it will pass
But how long is a faze and how long will it last
I've been knocked down so many times can I
always bounce back
Make my life colourful again get away from all this
black

ALARM BELL

You know me oh so well you can tell alls not well
Is it time to press the panic button and ring the
alarm bell
My eyes are so sore I could cry all the while
I feel so helpless it's hard to move an inch let
alone move a mile

Have things improved at all I don't really know
It doesn't feel like I'm getting anywhere I'm moving
so slow
Surely this isn't the way I'm always going to be
I don't know who I am anymore or whose the real
me

So many tablets I've taken and what have I gained
Just another chemical imbalance going around in
my brain
If I shout out loud would anyone hear me
Or am I trapped forever with my insanity

I used to be quite confident able to stand proud
and tall
But that's all gone now I've taken one almighty fall
Will I ever rise again and be that person once
more
Or forever shipwrecked miles away from life's
safety shore

BLANK EXPRESSION 2

All that I have is a blank expression on my face
All I have in my mouth is a bitter and nasty taste
If I could blame my illness on anyone would that
help me
The answer to that is no but it might help with the
uncertainty

I just feel so empty the future seems so bleak
I will always try to stay strong but do I appear
weak
I close my eyes try to escape for just a short time
The pain just seems to get worse it seems to blow
my mind

Why did this illness choose me what ever did I do
So many unanswered questions I don't have a
single clue
Would it help me if my future was mapped out
Would that give me strength give me more clout

What can I do to help myself to help myself get
better
Should I write it all down send myself a get well
letter
Just to be able to free myself from forever feeling
so low
Being allowed to move on with all systems on full
go

A GAMBLE WORTH TAKING

After fighting so hard for so very long
Things aren't going well so much is wrong
You won't hear me shout or start complaining
But a radical change is a gamble worth taking

I know there's a risk to everything we do
But I've got insight it's not like I haven't got a clue
It's just when your so depressed for ever feeling
low
You reach the point when you will give anything a
go

The support that I have is second to none
People I love and trust will tell me if I come
undone
I just need for the depression to lift
That's all I ask for just a simple gift

I know I've got my own faith so I will say another
prayer
Hopefully inch by inch step by step we will get
there
I will be able to see that flicker of light shining for
me
Slowly I will arrive at my life's destiny

WHAT'S ON YOUR MIND

You ask please tell me what's on your mind
Please understand it's hard to tell I'm trying to be
kind
It's difficult to put into words the darkness that I
feel
A feeling of despair, fear, and panic it's so very
real

I know your there for me and that means oh so
much
Your words and compassion your warmth care
and touch
Knowing that your fighting for me in my time of
despair
Please understand how grateful and thankful I am
because you care

The last 4 years have been such a turbulent time
I've done nothing wrong mental illness my only
crime
Let's hope it's nearly time to turn the corner and
fight back
To draw from the experience be thankful of what I
have rather than I lack

I've cried so many tears my emotions pushed to
the limit
But I will never give in to it throw in the towel or
submit
Because if there's one thing I can do that is to fight

So one day things will be better then I will feel alright

TURN BACK TIME

If I could turn back time would I change anything
I suppose that's just wishful thinking what good
would it bring
I would be carrying on working every hour god
sent
Cocooned in my own little world not really a gent

Having blinkered vision unaware of things around
me
Thinking only of myself that's how I know I would
be
Neglecting my family was something I didn't want
to do
But that was how it was a rethink was long
overdue

People I've met on this rollercoaster ride of mine
Have made me see things differently my soul
started to shine
When you look around you see people for what
they really are
Then my wounds begin to heal all that's left is the
scar

A reminder of that person that was once me
A person I thought I liked but I didn't really
So let time continue because it will never go back
Happy with the new me even though flawed but
not completed cracked

BAD NEWS

Events will unfold that's without a doubt a certainty
A feeling of fear takes a hold of me
You give me decisions to make options to choose
No silver lining to be found you give me bad news

I know it's not your fault and it's something you
have to do
But it tears me apart do you have a clue
How hard it is for me to make it through each day
So much hidden hurt, obstacles that are in my way

I wish that my future was planned out for me
Perhaps some of the fear would go and allow me
to be free
The uncertainty would go allow me to breath
I could then move on after a short time to grieve

So let things happen as quick as they can
Then I can think ahead and start to plan
Of my future and things I want from my life
No more looking back or living on the edge of a
knife

PHYSICAL WRECK

Once again I've gone to pieces once more a
physical wreck
I feel I've let you all down become a pain in the
neck
I'm sorry you see me shaking, sweating and crying
But sometimes I can't cover it up I don't like lying

It feels like a volcano about to explode
My brain can't take any more it's on complete
overload
So tired of being constantly depressed and so low
You can see the pain etched on my face the strain
shows

Any lift I get seems to last only for a few days
Then my mood drops back into a deep depressive
phase
It's like a vicious cycle I don't seem to be able to
break
It reaches a point that I've taken as much as I can
take

The depression beats me up tears me completely
apart
Like someone driving a stake straight through my
heart
But I dig deep inside draw on something from
within
No matter what this illness throws at me I will
never give in

BREAKING POINT

When you reach breaking point what do you do?
Do you decide to pack in or do you search for a
clue
A clue that gives you hope for you to carry on
No matter how hard it is try to take control of the
situation

Don't bottle things up because that does no good
Be honest and open tell people what you know
you should
It's hard if not impossible to pull through on your
own
Get a good network of support don't try to go it
alone

No matter how long it takes be assured things will
get better
Try not to be hard on yourself write yourself a
letter
One that speaks and reassures you when your
low
That given time you will get better confidence will
begin to show

So when your at breaking point make it your
turning point
Make sure you are in control and that your nose
isn't out of joint
Hang on in there better times will lie ahead

Tell yourself of all the good things and dreams you have in your head

SIDE EFFECTS

A tablet to help you get well it sounds easy
But the downside is the side effects they don't
please me
I read all the leaflets that come with the pills
But they scare me to death make me feel more ill

They read weight loss then next they read weight
gain
As the pounds pile on it adds to my pain
I'm told to watch my diet start to exercise more
I didn't ask for all of this I just wanted a cure

Some of the effects well you have to smile
If you believed all of them god you would run a
mile
Like for sleeping tablets it says these may make
you drowsy
It's hilarious really but somehow it doesn't surprise
me

So I will just carry on taking the medicine
Putting up with the down side again and again
I'm sure in the long term all will be well
Then all of the side effects can go to hell

HARD ON MYSELF

So many people say don't be so hard on yourself
But as times moved on I feel left on the shelf
It's so hard when you're stuck in such a rut
Depression always pulling me down like a kick in
the gut

I know I can cover it up have a smile on my face
It appears nothings wrong but I feel a disgrace
For being so ill and suffering for so very long
If I feel good for a while it soon goes very wrong

That's why I wish that I could be reborn
But I'm wise enough to know I've had too many
false dawns
All I ask for is a quality of life so that I can move
on
I know I'll never be completely cured but the battle
can be won

So I hear you say be proud of yourself how your
coping
I will try because I'm not sitting around feeling
sorry for myself and moping
Maybe I can use this to help me, help me move on
Then finally I will have some control of this crazy
situation

FINISHED (NOT YET)

When you've worked for so long but it's taken away
It eats away at you bit by bit day by day
You can't help and think of the person you used to be
Having to rediscover yourself find out who is the new me

It's like your hearts been ripped out and you wonder why
Many minutes, hours and days I break down and cry
I know it's no ones fault there's no one I can blame
So why am I full of guilt why do I feel so much shame

Do I take it as one door closing will another open
Can I pick myself up and become 10 out of 10
Finally being in control of this illness once and for all
To be happy and proud of myself standing upright and tall

So I'm far from finished nowhere near yet
I will come out stronger and wiser on that you can bet
Then in the future hopefully I can give something back

Rid myself of all the grey areas everything white and black

GAINS/LOSSES

When I look back over the last 4 years I've gained
and lost
I'm so much better as a human being but it's been
at a cost
You see my mental illness; bipolar disorder not
only affects me
But it rips right through the heart of my loving
family

It's so hard to explain to them what went wrong
And to be so ill for so very long
For them to see their dad break down and cry
It's their dad who's so ill how do you explain why

I suppose what is needed is for the stigma to go
Educate children at school because then they will
know
Things won't change straight away it will take time
But then we will be accepted by all after all we've
done no crime

It is my belief that people with mental illness are
just so real
There's no put up shield their emotion you can
touch and feel
So if we can all pull together and do all that we
can
Then we can start a mental illness get well plan

ONE MILLION EACH YEAR

One million people commit suicide each and every
year
Does that mean anything to you does it fill you
with fear
Or are you one of those who says "that's the easy
way out"
Just because it's mental health no one seems to
shout

Surely something has to change something has to
be done
A time for people's attitudes to alter a new dawn
begun
People can choose to ignore it but it's not going to
go away
Don't say I'll do something about it tomorrow do it
today

It's a fact that mental illness affects one in four
So no one is immune it knows no boundaries
that's for sure
So if you know someone who is mentally ill
Show them that you care if you don't well who will

No one knows what's round the corner or what will
be
It might just creep up on you like it happened to
me
So don't ignore it bury your head in the sand

Please show some compassion please try to understand

THOUGHTS IN YOUR HEAD

Racing thoughts spinning around inside of my head
Never ever slowing down jumbled sentences are said
Not one single thought ever seems to stay for too long
Everything seems so right I won't accept that I'm wrong

When the thoughts are racing their impossible to stop
Moving from idea to idea can these thoughts start to drop
The energy comes from somewhere there's never a need to rest
Some kind of super endurance some super mental test

Going to bed well that just seems a waste of time
I hear you say you look shattered but inside I feel so fine
It's at this stage that the mania is well and truly setting in
The feeling of being a super human being comes from somewhere within

Unless you've been there it's so very hard to explain
The feeling of ultimate ecstasy nothing to lose everything to gain

There's a funny side to it I think it helps to smile
But the humorous side doesn't last only for a short
while

ONE STEP

There's no miracle cure oh how I wish there was
one
I would bottle it up then share it with everyone
The trouble is when the illness is in the mind
There's no quick fix you have to take one step at a
time

Sometimes to take that one step is so very hard to
do
It seems to take for ever so long feeling blue
Sometimes it feels that you're stuck going
nowhere at all
Scared of moving another inch just waiting for the
next fall

You go so far then a hiccup and back to square
one
It feels like any progress you've made has come
completely undone
So when it gets tough dig deep never stop the
fight
One day you will win and things will turn out alright

Learn to be proud of yourself because you're not
to blame
Try not to hide away don't feel any shame
No matter how long it takes I promise you will
bounce back
Be proud of all the things that you have rather
than the things you lack

MOVE ON

Is this the time for me to move on
Learn to cope better with this illness this situation
Put all that I've learnt use it at will
My life no longer on hold even though I'm ill

Learn to use my bipolar experience pass it on to others
Let's have a united mental illness movement all sisters and brothers
By working together surely we can make things better
No more just sitting on the fence be a go getter

If everyone puts in just that extra 10%
Using each others knowledge then we can start to make a dent
To slowly break down barriers let the stigma go
Educate people teach them let their understanding grow

You may say this is wishful thinking but I don't think so
Bit by bit we can change things, progress will show
And gradually we with mental illness won't feel any shame
But why should we after all we're not to blame

WOULD YOU DARE SWAP WITH ME

You can look and stare at me you can say you
look well
But mental illness isn't always obvious it's hard to
tell
So how it feels I just wish you all could see
But I can promise you wouldn't dare swap with me

To feel depressed and so low for no reason at all
Trying to take all the blows but then bound to fall
Time and time again picking myself up off the floor
You see for this illness there is no cure

A cocktail of pills to try to get your mood stable
Otherwise it's up through the roof or under the
table
Pills to lift you up pills to bring you down
Pills to keep you stable an ever lasting merry go
round

So please feel free to swap with me for just one
day
Then you will have the insight to feel this way
Perhaps more than compassion you will show
And a change in people's attitudes can start to
flow

TO BE HIGH (JUST A BIT)

Being so depressed and low for so long now
But managing just to carry on through it somehow
I just wish I could be high just a bit
Not high as in totally out of control just a small hit

How nice it would be to be confident and so free
To be able to hold my head high the person I want
to be
To go out socially feeling happy not having to hide
No longer having the shame just feeling full of
pride

A high that stays at the feel good stage
Without it going overboard that dreaded manic
rage
I don't think I'm asking too much
Back to how I want to be not out of touch

To feel happy to walk round feeling free
Doing what I want what will be will be
I know this is a wish but it can come true
Oh God please let it happen it's long overdue

SO TIRED

So tired of fighting, so tired of battling on
But I'm never going to give up this fight will be won
I suppose it's easy to say but harder to do
Draw on all my support network I will pull through

It's been 4 years of hell and there's still more to go
Inch by inch I will move forward confidence will
slowing grow
It's been very hard on me, hard on my family too
Without them how would I survive I haven't a clue

They have seen this person they love crumble and
break
So many tears and varied emotions so real not
fake
Having had so much love, compassion and care
It gives hope and inspiration because their there

So as a person I've changed for the better it's true
Now an uplifting mood is long overdue
Then if I can help anyone that's what I will do
Move onwards and upwards start all fresh and
new

SUPPORT GROUP

When we first went to the support group we were full of fear
Taking that step through the door how would it be, no idea
But we were met by smiling faces and soon put at ease
Sit back and listen or join in if you please

It's so nice to know that your not on your own
Your not the only one with bipolar your not alone
Everyone has their own stories to tell
Of when they've been ill or how to try and stay well

For people with the illness and their carers too
Shared knowledge and experience will enlighten you
In no time at all the group will become your friend
If your life seems completely broken it could well start to mend

So if you've considered going to a group and thought no
Listen to my advice why not give it a go
It's proven they help so what can you lose
Start to learn more about bipolar the group's there if you choose

YOU'VE DONE SO WELL

I remember so well how ill you were a year ago
You had reached rock bottom you said you had
never been so low
I remember you were a mess shaking rock bottom
and down
But you sought help took the first steps to turn it
around

I remember when we met 4 years ago
You thought I was undercover staff I laughed and
said no
Over the weeks we became very good friends
When you meet where we met that friendship
never ends

Over the years we've chatted away so much
Opening up to each other making sure we stayed
in touch
So how you were a year ago it's hard to tell
But I'm proud of you because you've done so well

You are now so confident where before you were
a broken man
You've took control of your life you seem to have a
plan
I'm sure everything will turn out how you want it to
be
Be proud of yourself, know your own life's destiny

NO HELP

You say you don't need any help so why are you
here
You say you don't believe in medication is that fact
or just a fear
You say that everyone's against you that's simply
not true
I can see the anger in your eyes because you are
so blue

My own opinion is that you can't do it all on your
own
Family and friends support are what you need
when you're at home
Someone who knows you and will listen to what
you have to say
Friends that can help you get over any obstacles
in your way

So don't say you don't need any help you haven't
lost your pride
By seeking the right guidance is a plus something
you've tried
Many people who are mentally ill have isolated
themselves
But then they slip through the net and get left on
the shelf

So don't shut yourself off because it does no good
If it helps then every single one of us would

Hiding away hoping things would sort themselves out
But this would be naive who would hear us when we shout

ALWAYS GOT TIME

You seem to always have time for everyone you
see
When I've been really ill you've always talked to
me
There are things from my past which I've left
behind
You've never brought them up you've just been
kind

Your a credit to your profession if only all were like
you
I believe people would get better sooner, you
know just what to do
I have never seen you ignore anyone or turn them
away
Given them good advice or listen to what they say

With more like you we can get rid of the "us" and
"them"
So everyone gets a good service from the mental
health system
I know everyone can't be the same that's such a
shame
Rather than just being a NHS number you know
all our names

I'm so glad I know you because you're a wonderful
man
Pushing down boundaries doing all that you can
I can see things improving I know it will take time

But things will be done quicker with you doing fine

A REAL FRIEND

I've had so many friends over the years
Many have shared my laughter but few have seen
the tears
It's when you're in need that the cream raises to
the top
Some friends are scared of mental illness your
friendship didn't drop

You were there at the start when the mania set in
To start with it was funny it wasn't a crime or a sin
I felt on top of the world but this wasn't real
You were next to me it must have seemed so
surreal

Within a few days the point of laughter had gone
Everyone else knew something serious was wrong
except this one
So carted off to hospital for some reason I chose a
police car
You were in constant touch with my wife, a real
star

While in hospital you visited me on so many
occasions
Showing you cared; you listened and advised no
matter what the situation
If I was upset you would always make me smile
Some people go the extra inch you went the extra
mile

So one day I hope to return the favour, help you out
Call on me anytime if you need me just shout

FOUR YEARS AND COUNTING

If you told me how things would be I never would
have believed
You could have tried to tell me but it wouldn't have
been received
By me because for a while things felt so good
My life felt so great things going how they should

I was popular busy with lots of new things to do
I didn't see this illness creep up on me I wonder
did you
From feeling so confident I felt I could reach the
sky
It came on so quick but I soon went sky high

To me nothing seemed wrong I felt that I was King
No one could understand me or the upset it would
bring
It just felt that I had all the right things to say
From everything being fine it had all gone wrong
by the 7th day

You asked me to see a doctor I asked why I
wasn't ill
But everyone else knew I was I didn't listen until
My youngest daughter who was just 8 at the time
Said please go to the doctors daddy, I said OK
fine

So off we all went me my wife and 3 children

I told the doctor there's nothing wrong again and again
But he diagnosed me with manic depression
To me that meant nothing left me with a blank expression

Would I go to a psychiatric hospital hell no way
Or take tablets not a chance I heard myself say
So later that night I had to be sectioned
Led away taken to hospital like I had an infection

Now I had been "mentally ill" years ago 3 times in fact
But never diagnosed no knowledge at all information I lacked
So it was 4 years ago that this journey began
Even though it's been so very tough I'm a better man

Hopefully in the future things I've learnt I will pass on
If I can help someone who ends up in a similar situation
Maybe the stigma will start to shift out of the door
Because it's not a well known fact that mental illness affects 1 in 4

WAITING

Waiting to get better why does it take so long
I'm waiting for things to go right but they seem to go just wrong
I don't know what the future holds that's why I'm so scared
I've known this day would come I'm just not prepared

You say the pressure will be off and recovery will begin
Why do I feel so guilty bipolar disorder is my only sin
You see it's hard to bounce back up when I'm knocked down again
You say that I've looked fine to you but you can't see my internal pain

But you see I was born a fighter this is a fight I will not lose
I may be down nearly out on the ropes but to survive is what I choose
One day soon I will rise again back where I belong
A stronger, wiser, fitter man I pray it's not too long

I try not to think of the time that has gone as time that's been wasted
It's part of who I am now a new experience that I have tasted
Being in control is what I want surely that has to be my plan

Then I will know that I've arrived as a new born
man

www.ingramcontent.com/pod-product-compliance
Lightning Source LLC
Chambersburg PA
CBHW031159270326
41931CB00006B/338